Teaching the Moving Child

D0568598

Teaching the Moving Child

OT Insights that Will Transform Your K–3 Classroom

by

Sybil M. Berkey
Kirkland, Washington

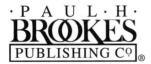

·P A U L·H·
BROOKES
PUBLISHING CO.®

Baltimore • London • Sydney

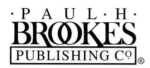

Paul H. Brookes Publishing Co.
Post Office Box 10624
Baltimore, Maryland 21285-0624
USA

www.brookespublishing.com

Copyright © 2009 by Paul H. Brookes Publishing Co., Inc.
All rights reserved.

"Paul H. Brookes Publishing Co." is a registered trademark
of Paul H. Brookes Publishing Co., Inc.

Manufactured in the United States of America by
Sheridan Books, Inc., Chelsea, Michigan.

Purchasers of *Teaching the Moving Child: OT Insights that Will Transform Your K–3 Classroom*
are granted permission to photocopy the blank forms in the text for educational purposes.
None of the forms may be reproduced to generate revenue for any program or individual.
Photocopies may only be made from an original book. *Unauthorized use beyond this privilege is
prosecutable under federal law.* You will see the copyright protection notice at the bottom of
each photocopiable page.

Library of Congress Cataloging-in-Publication Data

Berkey, Sybil M.
    Teaching the moving child : OT insights that will transform your K–3 classroom / by Sybil M.
    Berkey.
        p.   cm.
    Includes bibliographical references and index.
    ISBN-13: 978-1-59857-064-9 (pbk.)
    ISBN-10: 1-59857-064-1
    1. Readiness for school.   2. Motor ability in children.   3. Occupational therapy for children.
    I. Title.
    LB1132.B47   2009
    371.9'0472–dc22   2009024535

British Library Cataloguing in Publication data are available from the British Library.

2013   2012   2011   2010   2009

10   9   8   7   6   5   4   3   2   1

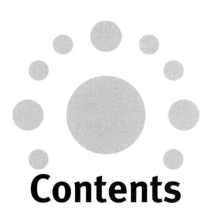

Contents

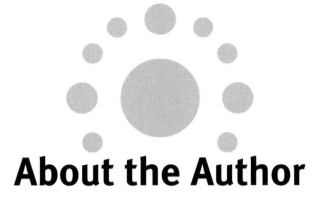

About the Author

Sybil M. Berkey, M.S., OTR, LOT, has served for more than 34 years in the field of occupational therapy, predominantly working as an occupational therapist in public schools. She has also served as an instructor at the University of Washington's School of Occupational Therapy and consulted for nursing care centers in the greater Seattle area.

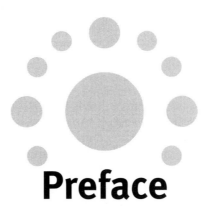

Preface

Teachers and occupational therapists (OTs) cross paths every day in the halls of American public schools. Our knowledge domains become linked, to some degree, through collaboration regarding the educational needs of struggling students, through in-service opportunities, through informal discourse, and through the modeling of our skill bases as we work in the classroom and present our evaluation findings in the many meetings we attend together.

Currently, more than 35,000 occupational therapy practitioners, nearly one third of the professional workforce, are employed in school settings (American Occupational Therapy Association, 2006) under the provisions of the Individuals with Disabilities Education Improvement Act of 2004 (IDEA 2004). Historically, the role of the OT in the educational environment has been defined under the umbrella of special education. Services to children have primarily been reserved for those who are found, through the formal initial evaluation process, to be eligible for special education and the necessary related services designed to ameliorate the adverse educational impact of disability or developmental delay. Occupational therapists, trained in the art and science of enhancing children's engagement in the meaningful ecological *occupations* demanded in their role as students, thus collaborate daily with teachers and caregivers.

That OTs are mandated to work in the public schools is testament to the understanding that dysfunction in motor ability, sensory processing, or independence in the functional performance tasks of work, play, leisure, and social encounters can create obstacles to a child's learning and successful educational outcome. The relationship between teachers and OTs, however, is changing with the encouragement of the U.S. Department of Education, toward the implementation of new approaches to problem solving, including response to intervention, and positive behavioral supports. Such pre-referral prevention and remediation will increase collaborative efforts to enhance the ability of *general* education to meet the needs of students who struggle in school.

Awareness of the foundations of educational and occupational therapy theories, with their perspectives of learning as embedded in the context of environment and constrained by the demands of learning tasks, should inevitably draw teachers and OTs closer together in a mutual understanding of the work of the child within the educational setting. The handwriting process, for example, cannot be described as singly cognitive or language or motor, and its instruction and remediation must address all domains.

All professionals will benefit from an appreciation of the functional interplay between student factors, environmental components, and task demands, as agents for change (for better or for worse), and the possibility that excessive demand may drive adaptation toward compromised function. Teachers can become frustrated and disheartened when a child who struggles in the classroom may not be recommended for occupational therapy services by the evaluation team. A mutual understanding of the student–environment–task interplay can hasten a more coherent analysis of the problem, inspire early intervening services, and diminish the assumption of disability or developmental delay.

My reasons for writing this book, however, both encompass and transcend policy and theory and are, in addition, practical and personal. First, I find that K–3 teachers—among the most ardent, engaged, and energetic of my colleagues—are simply very thirsty for a greater comprehension of the sensory and motor foundations of learning and the reasonable expectations of classroom performance in critical areas such as handwriting and attending behavior. Second, despite burgeoning brain-based research by neuroscientists, published implications for methodology in the classroom, and constructivist assumptions about learning and developmentally appropriate teaching practice, the contemporary compression of the primary (K–3) general education curriculum comes, in my observation, at an unacceptable cost to the playful nature, motor proficiency, self-regulatory capacity, and functional performance of our youngest learners.

Third, I am observing signs of stress in young students, ranging from the rejection of writing tasks to behavior that is generally challenging, and these signs are not often attributed by policy makers to the increasing academic and social-emotional demands of the modern curriculum. Primary teachers, though, are often intuitive about this link, and many have voiced concern that the early curriculum is biologically inappropriate for 5- to 8-year-old children. Late in the last school year, having suspected a disquieting trend, I reviewed the characteristics of my caseload. As a member of the evaluation team, I am routinely called upon to evaluate the sensorimotor and occupational performance of young students who are struggling in the classroom. Of the many elementary-age children referred for initial occupational therapy evaluations, I calculated that, to my apprehension but not to my great surprise, 100% were little boys—*one hundred percent!* Considering that many children (girls and boys alike) are found to have typical sensorimotor skills despite an inability to meet performance demands in the classroom, a large red flag should be raised on their behalf.

Fourth, I am convinced that, given a mutual understanding of growing cognition and learning as embodied processes, the sensory and motor capacities of young children can and should be considered as allies to learning across all domains, and not simply as kinesthetic strategies in service to a particular learning style. Rather, there should exist a fluid approach to providing opportunities for sensorimotor learning, and natural movement should be engaged to mediate all learning in ways that language or linguistic understandings cannot accomplish alone. The child's natural energies can and should be recruited more effectively to enhance self-regulation and social-emotional competence, and to ameliorate academic stress within an increasingly rigorous curriculum. The more challenging the K–3 curriculum becomes, the more still become the bodies of young children, who, by nature, are wiggly, chatty, often off-task and off-topic, and whose movements and learning are inexorably linked to the great benefit of their cognitive development and academic success. As K–3 teachers learn more about the sensory and motor development of children, and consider alternative strategies for the presentation of core instruction within the framework of the student–environment–task balance, the more they are likely to teach children who are alert, relaxed, focused, and ready to learn.

I have chosen to direct these materials particularly to my K–3 general education colleagues, since so many of the foundations of functional educational performance are established at this level, and secondarily to my OT colleagues, who might gain a greater appreciation of the influences of educational theory and practice on their own work with young students, and for whom *educational relevance* might assume a more precise significance. This is not principally a book about the remediation of disability, although information regarding children with special needs, particularly in Chapters 4 and 5, will be integrated under the assumption that all children in the classroom are the primary responsibility of the general education teacher. (And also because, as an OT, I simply cannot help it!) Nor is it chiefly a collection of specific classroom strategies, although a number will be offered. Rather, as I have always preferred in my collaborations with teachers and parents, I have chosen to frame the principles underlying occupational performance and the interplay between student, environmental, and task constraints in support of core instruction. Thus, the internalization of these principles will permit others to create and implement creative and effective approaches that I might never have considered myself.

It is my hope that this book will reawaken an awareness of the multiple developmental components of learning; begin the process of professional knowledge sharing (in this case, from OT to teacher); begin to prevent many preventable learning obstacles; inform the collaborative process in schools; and frame the collaborative efforts of teachers and OTs based on shared understandings of the interplay between student factors, environmental elements, and task demand. Finally, I hope to address many of the astute and heartfelt questions that come my way each year from so many devoted educators, and I hope that the student–environment–task framework will enable the teacher–OT connection to thrive for the benefit of kids.

REFERENCES

American Occupational Therapy Association. (2006). *Workforce trends in occupational therapy*. Retrieved December 20, 2007, from http://www.aota.org/search.aspx?SearchPhrase=workforce+trends

Individuals with Disabilities Education Improvement Act (IDEA) of 2004, PL 108-446, 20 U.S.C. §§ 1400 *et seq.*

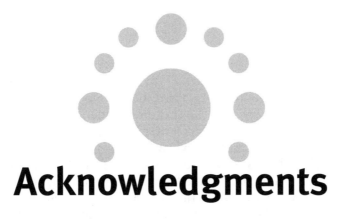

Acknowledgments

Brilliant and a man of few words, my Dad was, above all else, playful and inventive to the end of his life. Raised on a farm in South Dakota, he earned a reputation as mischievous and curious, a combination that earned him both tribulation and notoriety. I still have the photograph, circa 1935, of him with his brothers as they found a way to short-cut their chores—by shucking peas through my Grandmother's wringer wash machine. That was the curious and inventive part. The curious and mischievous part got him into big trouble when, in the middle of the Great Depression, he electrocuted my Grandfather's prize sow, Susie, causing her to lose much of her weight and most of her value.

Here's how he did it: Enthralled with his father's new electric fencing, and while experimenting with science, Dad carefully placed one prong of a pitchfork on the active fence and another prong on the nose of one of Susie's piglets. What better entertainment for a young farm boy as the piglet jumped, squealed, and scampered away, surprised but unscathed. But then, mental wheels turning, Dad raised the bar on science and invited an unsuspecting Susie over to participate. Problem was, she had a metal ring through her nose, and when electric fence met pitchfork met ring, Susie jumped and squealed like her piglets, but didn't run anywhere. She nearly dropped dead, and Dad spent the remainder of his summer rolling the weak and listless sow over in her pen, positioning her so that her piglets could nurse until weaned.

Throughout my childhood, Dad's antics were a delight to me and my siblings and, at times, a trial to my long-suffering mother. I always declined to take part in the ghost stories, but secure in maternal arms, I loved to watch Dad scare the living daylights out of my older brother and sister. As they held hands around the dining room table, the house dark and still, Dad would conjure up an invisible spirit, proving its presence by surreptitiously rocking the table with his knees. Now in a heightened state of trepidation, my edgy but willing siblings were sent upstairs to hunt for the unearthly visitor. Then my favorite part: Dad bangs the ceiling with a broom handle, and brother and sister race screaming down the stairs, breathless and ready to do it again.

At the dinner table, we heard nightly chapters in the "true-life story" of Totem Pole Pete. The enchanting tale went on for months as we learned how Dad chased and eventually captured the notorious outlaw in the desert Southwest. He even showed us the scar on his side, where the bullet from Pete's blazing six-gun pierced Dad's flesh in one spot and exited from another. It wasn't until years later, when I asked my uncle about the injury, that I learned how Dad was, in actual fact, wounded while climbing over a barbed wire fence on their childhood farm. I never told him that I knew.

I could go on. There was the time he strained his shoulder while simulating how one would land safely after parachuting out of an airplane. Or the time he zipped his jacket over the top of his head and pretended to be the "Headless Horseman." While he set out to entertain his grandchildren, the episode is better remembered for the major black and blue lump which rose prominently on Dad's forehead after he ran smack into the kitchen cabinet. And one of my personal favorites: the time during my brief phase of adolescent rebellion when I brought home my first and only D grade. Dad held the test paper out at arms length, cocked his head in mock concentration, and turned the paper on its side until the D rotated just so. Then, proclaiming "Oh… an A!" he handed it back to me with that little sly smile and never said another word.

My Dad was a lifelong kindergartner, prizing the same qualities in himself and his children that we should value and preserve in our youngest students. He was, as a result, the most skilled and effective teacher I ever had, placing the "grade" in its proper perspective and elevating my love of learning to a level of self-sustainability. He left this world way too early, but characteristically, he left it in the midst of play. Who better to acknowledge as the inspiration for this book than the man who so thoroughly understood the joy of childhood and the great worth in questioning and seeking and learning.

In addition, I wish to thank Terri Mendenhall and Megan Elliott for their technical expertise and artistic assistance, and mostly for their gracious willingness to help whenever I called. Thanks also to Lynn Armstrong, Heather Frazier, and Colleen McAlerney for their generosity in sharing photographs and professional expertise. Special thanks to the Chen, Kent, Nelson, and Shadbakht families, whose generosity has given life to this project.

To David and Cale

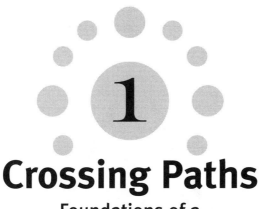

Crossing Paths

Foundations of a
Collaborative Prevention Model

To meet the promise of success for all children at the kindergarten to grade 3 (K–3) level, school-based professionals, including teachers and occupational therapists (OTs), must pool their perspectives and understandings in the educational domain. It is the opportune time to develop new paradigms for collaboration on the design, delivery, and evaluation of core instruction at the base of a prevention model and on the interventions that target the challenges of the struggling child. Toward this end, school-based professionals should first prioritize, articulate, and agree on the terms of their collaborative efforts.

1. They must recognize the shared operational inheritance of professional theory, educational policy, and practice.
2. They must recommit to the multiple foundations of learning and share their unique knowledge bases as they contribute to the education of young children and the prevention of learning barriers.
3. They must embrace an integrated and holistic or all systems approach to educational policy and planning founded on generalized, high-quality, research-based methodologies that are derived from a range of expertise.
4. They must frame their collaborations with the three components of educational performance, which include student factors, environmental components, and task demands (see Figure 1.1).

Teachers and OTs share a common context in the public schools, and the professional approaches of both are shaped by a variety of interrelated factors and influences. Theory that grounds one quietly affects the other. In addition, federal and state policies decisively frame both. Contemporary education issues draw them closer together in a mutual expectation of *best practices* for students.

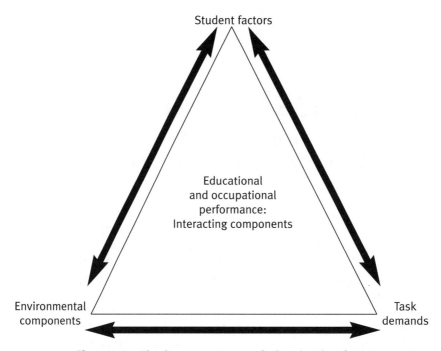

Figure 1.1. The three components of educational performance.

As often as they cross paths, however, the undercurrent of common perspective is rarely explicit in their collaborations and has the potential to be more influential than seems apparent. As federal and state educational mandates call teachers and OTs toward a system of prevention and problem solving, the most effective services at the level of *core instruction* will combine the theory, expertise, and practice methods of all members of the education team.

Core instruction, also called *universal interventions* or *primary supports*, is at the base of a multi-tiered service delivery model now being used by many states and local school districts. The Individuals with Disabilities Education Improvement Act (IDEA) of 2004 (PL 108-446) calls for struggling and at-risk students to be supported with problem-solving approaches known as response to intervention (RTI) and positive behavioral support (PBS), which provide scientific, research-based early intervening services designed to prevent academic failure and ameliorate the impact of at-risk performance (Nanof, 2007). Implementation of these initiatives first considers curriculum and its delivery and seeks to provide immediate strategies for any child struggling with the demands of core instruction and children who are at risk of requiring more intensive specially designed instruction. This new thinking about what supports successful educational outcome has begun to distance us from the old perspective of a singular question: "What is going wrong with the student?" It has adjusted the relationship among team members and is calling the OT away from a specific role in "fixing" impairment or remediating dysfunction toward a more comprehensive partnership in the education of all children.

The RTI model, patterned on prevention–intervention models in public health, was designed to specifically address criticisms of the *wait-to-fail* system of identifying specific learning disabilities (National Research Center on Learning Disabilities, 2006). It is applied in the field of education as a process designed to *prevent* chronic learning problems. Quality research-based core classroom instruction is at the base (Tier 1) of this multi-tiered model and is provided in the general education classroom by the general education teacher. Core instruction is assumed to provide appropriate learning experiences for all students, the vast majority of whom, as research has demonstrated, will perform at expectation. *Targeted interventions,* which are at the second tier of the model, are directed toward an anticipated 15% of students who are identified during a regular screening process, continue to have difficulty with core instruction, and require alternative methodologies or supplemental tutoring programs designed by school-based problem-solving teams (National Association of State Directors of Special Education, 2006). The final or third tier of the RTI model is focused on those students (evidence predicts approximately 5%) who, after frequent progress monitoring, continue to struggle with targeted interventions and are referred for *intensive intervention* or special education services. When implementing RTI, general educators, special educators, and specialist or support staff (including OTs) are encouraged to collaborate to provide screening, monitor progress, and provide effective instructional strategies in a coherent and seamless system *prior to* special education referral.

The effectiveness of core instruction, however, which is often based on constructivist educational theory (discussed later in this chapter), appears to be under siege in the current climate of the standards movement and the consequent compression of the K–3 curriculum. School readiness, developmentally appropriate practice (DAP), and the aspiration of a child-centered approach become less practical as conceptual frameworks in a system that seems to tilt its focus and favor toward benchmarks and grade-level expectations.

Theoretical underpinnings and evidence-based practice for both educators and OTs value the interplay among student, environment, and task. More than ever, the contextualized approach to instruction for successful academic outcome is critical in the educational setting. A developmental perspective alone is of limited value because the chronological and developmental diversity of the youngest learners broadens the ability range of the typical group of 5- to 8-year-olds and precludes a single instructional approach. The cognitive, social, physical, and sensory elements of both environment and academic task weigh heavily in the formula for optimal educational performance. Despite theoretical heritage and attempts to interweave the critical components of recommended practice, observable stress behaviors documented in school-age children are testimony to a precarious balance of the student–environment–task interplay.

THE COLLABORATIVE FRAMEWORK: STUDENT, ENVIRONMENT, AND TASK

The best educational outcomes for young children, sought through attention to the growing intellect, are equally balanced with the central social-emotional foundations and self-regulatory capacities of the learning child. Stillness is balanced with movement in service to attention and action, logic and creativity, and memory and motivation. Learning tasks offer the appropriate challenge. The educational environment offers stimulation through the senses, balanced with elements that calm and organize the child for optimal learning readiness.

In contemplating the three components of the student–environment–task framework, several things become apparent. First, both teachers and OTs are often underinformed regarding the full extent of the integration between academic and neurodevelopmental or sensorimotor components of educational task demand. (This is explained further in discussions of handwriting and sensory processing in Chapters 4 and 5.) Second, the interplay among student, environment, and task characteristics is typically undervaluated in instructional design and in the assessment of educational outcome. Third, a mismatch among the three contributors to successful outcome not only plays a role in children's frustration in school, but also is a factor in mislabeling many children as ineffectual learners (Eide & Eide, 2006). Fourth, evidence is pointing to the likelihood that many learning challenges are more correctible than once thought (Melillo & Leisman, 2004). Fifth, it is hoped that systematic attention to the multitude of interacting factors will alert all education team members to the importance of balance among the critical elements of successful performance, as well as integrate those elements productively for optimal educational outcomes and the prevention of learning obstacles.

A critical review of the educational environments and tasks both precede and accompany an assessment of student factors for the child who cannot meet expectations. Initial careful design of the environment and heightened awareness of the multiple developmental components of task are preventive at the level of core instruction. Thought processes of curriculum planning, evaluation of the effectiveness of current instructional methodologies, and strategic planning at the level of targeted interventions all draw on the combined expertise of team members whose common perspectives become explicit through collaboration.

Student Factors

Professionals in the education environment are trained to observe and evaluate the specific skills of the child, whether cognitive, academic, sensorimotor, perceptual, linguistic, attentional, or social-emotional. They have at their disposal a great number of criterion- and norm-referenced assessment measures in addition to maintaining work portfolios and taking daily notes about ability, behavior, and progress. They document children's performance skills and note their work and self-regulatory patterns. They assign a numeric or descriptive value to everything from phonemic awareness to pencil grasp. They attend parent conferences and evaluation feedback meetings and report on IQs, academic grade equivalents, developmental motor ages, and peer interactions. They learn a lot about the children and know that the unique abilities of each child play prominently in the formula for successful educational outcome. However, student characteristics or factors do not operate in isolation and cannot independently explain the reason for success or struggle on any given educational task. Whether designing curriculum or instructional methods or problem solving for strategic intervention, two other elements of educational performance—environmental components and task demand—must be considered. Each of these elements is discussed in the following sections.

Environmental Components

Many educators and therapists have found that a young child can perform independently in one environment but may require support for the same activity in another. Teachers sometimes question a therapist who claims that a child produces beautiful handwriting in the intervention room when legibility is elusive in the classroom. It is a common phenomenon and is related to the interplay of task and environment. Classrooms are inherently busy, as measured by any sensory standard. Walls are colorful, vibrant, and simultaneously display work samples, alphabet strips, posters, rules of behavior, word boards, and calendars. Mobiles hang from ceilings, and materials and manipulatives are stacked in bins. Cubbies are bursting with papers, coats, and snacks. Learning centers are fully equipped, computers are in use, and furniture is placed just so. In some classrooms, bare space is hard to find. All sensory channels are heavily enriched in the K–3 physical environment. Music plays, little voices escalate, and chimes signal a transition in the auditory surroundings. Lighting is typically fluorescent and can sometimes flash for attention to task. Little hands have a multitude of tactile experiences, and little bodies are in close proximity.

It is important to remember, however, that there is more to environment than the physical space. Culture and language are overarching. The curriculum itself is part of the environment as it is presented by the teacher and visibly displayed on the walls. Every adult in the classroom is part of it. Voice quality, temperament, and mannerisms are part of it. The pace of the day is part of it. Peers share it. Every transition changes it. Environments are inside, outside, open, or compact, all with a unique set of demands. Whatever the environment, we tend to underestimate its impact in the educational performance of the child in school.

Task Demand

The final element of educational performance is task demand. This may be explained by considering that a teacher looks through "educational lenses." By doing so, the teacher is most cognizant of the academic or cognitive task demands, which are often articulated in published learning requirements and grade-level expectations. A first grader, for example, may be expected to write several sequenced sentences. The end product will be quite visible, but the process is laden with hidden task demands. What is the sequence of steps in the task? What is the time allotment for task completion? What are the vocabulary and orthographic loads? The teacher, however, may be less attuned to many equally essential task components, which may be readily evident to an OT. What, for example, are the tools and materials the child is required to manipulate? What kind of paper is provided (lined or unlined)? Does the furniture support optimal posture? What level of fine motor ability is required? What are the sensory challenges? The OT must also seek to understand the academic task demands that bear on a child's handwriting legibility or weigh on his or her physical self-management.

In attending more closely to these components of performance and in drawing from diverse expertise to examine their individual characteristics, the education team will become increasingly alert to the interactions among student, environment, and task and the consequent influence, either negative or supportive, that each has on the others. Requiring careful planning and anticipation, the subtle changes in relative interaction that occur with variations in environment or task demand will become more apparent. Why, for example, might a particular child's aggressive behavior more likely erupt during an all-school assembly or when he or she is waiting in line? Why can another child weave a fantastic oral tale but struggle to put words to paper? Which student factors warn us to anticipate hesitation from one child when his or her peers are happily engaged in a group activity? What external supports will enhance the sustained attention of a child who notices even minor changes in the visual environment?

Having discussed the primary collaborative framework of the student–environment–task interplay, it is appropriate in the interest of mutual understanding to review a number of the common elements of school-based practice derived from the educational and occupational therapy professions. Such a sampling explores some of the mutual influences grounding the work of teachers and OTs whose common context is the educational environment and whose collective goals include a broadening awareness of the components of educational performance, an improvement of educational outcome, a reduction in the need for remediation, and an amelioration or elimination of sources of stress for the young child in school.

THEORY IN CONTEXT: EDUCATION

Educational theory finds root in basic philosophy concerning the nature of reality and existence (metaphysics); the theory of knowledge (epistemology); the formation of values, ethics, and aesthetics (axiology); and the rules of valid critical thinking (logic) (Pulliam & Van Patten, 1999). It is further sifted through schools of educational philosophy, including idealism, realism, pragmatism, and behaviorism, with each having a distinguishing rationale.

From these various schools of thought, many fundamental questions have arisen to challenge the essential architecture of educational foundation, function, operation, and curriculum. Do the public schools function to socialize children as citizens of their particular society or equip them to develop a worldview? Do they teach them to discern a truth that is absolute or to construct a personal reality based on the integration of new knowledge and unique experience? Is the classroom child centered, knowledge centered, or subject centered? Is the classroom traditional or constructivist? Is the teacher an expert or facilitator? Is the content basic or flexible? Are the students passive or active? Are the children ready or hurried?

As systematic, scientific, and accountable as education is now becoming, the history of its theory is rich with the gritty lives of great and influential thinkers who developed new ideas and chose bold departures, lost or gained confidence and favor, battled personal demons, and meticulously observed the world of their day. From the writings and biographies of these intellectual guardians, common conceptual threads can be traced forward to the modern public classroom.

Contemporary pedagogy is heir to the celebrated works of Jean-Jacques Rousseau (Damrosch, 2005), John Dewey (Campbell, 1995; Martin, 2002), Jean Piaget (Evans, 1973; Piaget, 1975), and Lev Vygotsky (Daniels, Cole, & Wertsch, 2007). From just these four giants of educational theory, modern classrooms can assimilate a value on the means of the acquisition of knowledge over conventional memorization and discipline, place a priority on action-based learning that is derived from a child's own natural impulse to learn, teach from the child's place of readiness, influence the environment and task in a child's construction of knowledge, and, indeed, promote the foundational theory of constructivist education.

The works of Lev Vygotsky are enjoying resurgent application in modern educational research and practice and merit particular exploration. Children's growth, according to Vygotsky, is mediated through intellectual tools, such as language, that they acquire from their culture and that they use in negotiating with and learning from more capable caregivers and peers (Bakhurst, 2007). The *zone of proximal development* (ZPD), a frequently applied concept, continues to be used heavily in both instruction and educational assessment (Bakhurst, 2007; Del Río & Álvarez, 2007). ZPD acknowledges the child's capacities from two perspectives. First, all children are in command of a core of completed development, which encompasses those tasks and problems that can be accomplished or solved independently and decisions that can be made without assistance. Yet, completed development is only a partial picture and does not reveal the range of more complex tasks that the child is capable of tackling when provided with guided instruction—*scaffolding*—in the form of leading questions, verbal or physical cues, or hints. With scaffolding, the child is drawn beyond his or her independent ability, and *potential* performance is revealed (Daniels, 2007; Haywood & Lidz, 2007). Thus, the ZPD represents the discrepancy between the level of capacity that is reached independently and the level that is reached with assistance from others. In this zone, learning and development are dynamically engaged. Scaffolding within the ZPD is not equivalent to task analysis for skill acquisition, nor is it a fruitless transmission of knowledge from learned to learner. It is, rather, a cooperative and collaborative conceptual interchange characterized by active participation in the learning community. Education teams increasingly encounter Vygotsky's concepts in current educational publications and bring their influence to the table during collaborations.

CONSTRUCTIVISM

Deriving from the works of the early theorists, particularly Piaget, and bearing scrutiny in learning research (Brooks & Brooks, 2001; DeVries, Zan, Hildebrandt, Edmiaston, & Sales, 2002), the theory of *constructivism* has significantly influenced the modern classroom in methodology, teacher and child roles, use of materials and activities, assessment, and classroom environment and structure. Constructivism holds that meaning is attached to learning when children are able to link new knowledge with prior experience and understanding (Henson, 2001; Piaget, 1975). Learning in the constructivist model inherently involves self-reorganization as the student resolves discrepancies between current personal perceptions and new insights within the social environment (Fosnot, 1996). The teacher in this model is a facilitator rather than an expert information provider who plans purposefully to enable the child's personal connections. A priority on scaffolding and student problem solving to facilitate understanding brings nontraditional approaches into the classroom. These may include small-group activities and integrated learning through the core curriculum. Both thematic curriculum or interdisciplinary units and project-based learning support constructivist education (Henson, 2001).

DeVries et al. (2002) offer seven principles of constructivist teaching. First is the creation of an atmosphere of cooperation and respect within which the child is encouraged to practice the self-regulation of behavior and is safe to participate and experiment with the construction of ideas. Second, the interests of the children, based on the teacher's careful observation and on the children's own questions, provide the foundation for *enticing activities* to promote learning. Opportunity for choice making draws attention to emerging interests. Third, teaching style changes with the type of knowledge elicited. The child struggling with the relationship of physical objects might be encouraged with leading questions. Errors in logical-mathematical reasoning might instead be addressed with leading experiences in which children are guided to revise and reconstruct their knowledge. Fourth, curriculum content with a focus on *big ideas* challenges open inquiry, leads to new insights, provokes curiosity, and sustains interest. Fifth, constructivist practice is child centered in the sense that children do the thinking as active participants in the learning process. They are not passive, and neither is the teacher whose interventions are artfully modified to draw the child toward greater awareness. The teacher first probes for current understanding and then creates just enough disequilibrium and contradiction to highlight a problem and begin the process of solution finding. Sixth, in-depth exploration is made possible with the allotment of sufficient time. Finally, the seventh principle is that teaching is linked to ongoing assessment of children's knowledge and to the effectiveness of the curriculum.

Constructivist teaching does not obligate the elimination of all didactic approach. The construction of new insights should take place seamlessly within projects or during more traditional group discussions and reflect the *way* children learn, regardless of the activity (DeVries et al., 2002). This educational model, however, has significant implications for the balance of student, environment, and task. The observer of the constructivist classroom will notice that even the arrangement of desks is designed to promote the collaboration of students who are naturally inclined to scaffold new understandings for each other. The special educator will be aware of the complexity of social thinking inherent in constructivist methods. The OT will weigh the educational costs and benefits of moving a child further from the group for the maintenance of sensory-based attention and learning readiness. Everyone on the team will address the unique needs of children based on a shared understanding of the theoretical source of classroom strategies and the rationale for classroom configuration, pace, and activity choice.

As theoretical and practical foundations are shared across professions, possible learning barriers are exposed. Project-based learning, for example, can abound with sensory encounters that may be intolerable to children with sensory processing disorder. Integrated curriculum content may inadvertently sacrifice essential rehearsal on discrete motor skills, particularly in the area of handwriting. The ZPD can be quite narrow for children with disabilities, and OTs often and necessarily design scaffolded instruction that is out of sync with the learning level of the classroom as a whole. Only shared perspective and informed collaboration will bring awareness to the team and ensure the likelihood of successful educational outcomes for all children within the context of the constructivist educational model.

OCCUPATIONAL THERAPY THEORY

Occupational therapy as a professional field of practice visibly entered allied health care in the early 20th century to provide services for the wounded soldiers of World War I. The heroine of this time, Eleanor Clarke Slagle, entered the nascent profession and began *habit training* classes, which used daily occupations to reeducate the lost or ineffectual *habits of living* for people with disabilities and those who had been injured in order to return them to a level of personal and financial independence. She rose quickly in the field and was instrumental in shaping the core values of the discipline, promoting legislative support, and launching schools and departments of occupational therapy across the United States (Quiroga, 1995).

The Education for All Handicapped Children Act of 1975 (PL 94-142), predecessor to IDEA 2004, provided a natural entry for OTs into the public schools, which now employ nearly one third of the OT work force (American Occupational Therapy Association, 2006). Similar to education, occupational therapy is both science and art, drawing pedagogically on such fields as anatomy, physiology, neurology, kinesiology, and human occupation, but also on the reasoning, creative capacities, and interpersonal proficiency of the therapist.

Educators will find immediate compatibility in the foundations of occupational therapy in such concepts as activity, occupation, context, and relevance. The daily activities of the student, those goal-directed actions required in the context of the educational environment, are of mutual concern to both professionals and can be as broad as learning and playing or as specific as handwriting. Every activity presents a unique combination and level of cognitive, language, attentional, movement, emotional, and sensory load, and each one appeals differently to the capacities and motivations of the child.

Guided by the natural drive to engage, as well as personal interests, needs, and choices, students transform activity into occupation that has meaning in their own lives. Occupation, then, continues to be the core principle of the profession, which supports the *occupational performance* of the child. Occupational performance occurs through the dynamic interaction among personal factors, environmental components, and task demands (American Occupational Therapy Association, 2008). In the school environment, collaboration among teachers and other education team members elevates the ability to analyze occupational performance and enable children's successful participation in, and execution of, school-related occupations from hanging up a coat to writing a coherent paragraph. It is the role of the OT to enable the child's participation in the occupations of school, and it is the art of both the OT and the teacher to choose methodology, materials, and practices, as well as to build rapport, which supports participation in those activities requisite in the school environment that may be neither the child's primary choice nor favored interest.

The importance of context and environment cannot be underestimated in the concept of occupation as meaningful to the child. Again, schools are rich with elements of social, cultural, physical, instructional, and technological environments. Children play and learn in the context of relationships with adults and peers and interact with other children and teachers of diverse ethnic and cultural backgrounds. They learn within the curricular and instructional context. They move in a variety of physical environments, including classroom, playground and gymnasium, cafeteria, music class, and computer lab, each presenting unique physical, academic, and sensory challenges to the child's participation. Mini environments exist even within the classroom itself and change constantly as the activity is individual or group based or carried out at the table or on the floor.

It is, in fact, the context that distinguishes the role of clinical and school-based OTs. In the private clinic, the OT is free to address any life domain that is important to the needs of the child and family in any context. In the educational environment, however, the OT, who is providing a service primarily related to special education, is mandated to assist the eligible student to participate in those occupations that are *educationally relevant* and to support the student's ability to access and benefit from the curriculum. Furthermore, OTs in the public schools provide occupational therapy services, although they anecdotally report requests to "do" sensory integration or handwriting instruction.

Frames of reference reflect a functional perspective and aid the therapist to "shift from theory into practice" (Kramer & Hinojosa, 1999, p. 3). Thus, sensory integration, for example, is one of several frames of reference and is applied when the child's ability to process sensory information does not serve his or her ability to respond adaptively to the demands of the educational environment nor to meet the occupational expectations of school (Kimball, 1999). Based on a comprehensive team evaluation, the OT chooses frames of reference that will best address the needs of the child and those occupations that are ecologically important at that particular time and within the context of the school environment.

Educational and occupational therapy theories represent primary sources of modern pedagogical practice and occupational performance, and awareness of their basics is more than an exercise in academics or history. Such awareness represents a shared operational inheritance unique to school-based professionals and is an essential link between the work of teachers and OTs as they serve the needs of students. It informs the collaborative process through the shared theoretical assumption of the student–environment–task interplay and challenges the need for knowledge sharing across professions.

Without a mutual understanding at this most basic level, it is unlikely that OTs would be aware of the implications of constructivist methodologies on their own practice with children in the public schools. Conversely, teachers are more likely to appreciate the modifications and accommodations recommended for children with disabilities when OTs are able to describe the influence of specific strategies on such learning constructs as motor competency, self-regulation, and attention.

SCHOOL READINESS AND
DEVELOPMENTALLY APPROPRIATE PRACTICE

Equally influential regarding the education of young children have been the concepts of *school readiness* and *developmentally appropriate practice* (DAP). In a 2005 policy report, the National Institute for Early Education Research (NIEER) comprehensively addressed diverse issues surrounding readiness (Ackerman & Barnett, 2005). It reiterated that chronological age is no longer the sole determinant of kindergarten eligibility, which has become more complex in consideration of increasing knowledge of child development, emerging measurable indicators of school readiness, diversity of prekindergarten experience, socioeconomic status, familial language, preparedness of schools to receive children with diverse backgrounds and abilities, and trends regarding increasing academic standards and delayed school start.

NIEER surveyed all state statutes regarding age eligibility for kindergarten and found that children are required to reach the age of 5 no later than October 16 in three fourths of U.S. states. (September is the predominant eligibility month [Ackerman & Barnett, 2005].) The institute concluded that school readiness is increasingly perceived as a problem issue based on the fact that nearly 30 years ago approximately 50% of school districts enrolled children whose fifth birthday fell as late as January. Whereas evidence regarding the merit of *redshirting* (holding children back) is mixed, approximately 7% of parents across the country delay entrance for their age-eligible children by at least 1 year, a trend that is more common for boys than girls. Given the variability of development, the maturational levels of children can thus be expected to reflect a 4-year spread among same-age peers by age 6 (Healy, 2004). NIEER further reported on teacher and parent perceptions of school readiness, preschool experience as it influences readiness, and urban and/or rural differences in school preparedness for children. As a policy recommendation, NIEER discourages delayed kindergarten entry. Instead, the institute encourages the application of factors that enhance both child and school readiness and DAP, which, if effective, should render delayed start a rare occurrence.

Also in 2005, the National School Readiness Indicators Initiative (2005), a 17-state partnership, published the results of their collaboration on the issue with the articulated goals of defining terminology and determining related measurable indicators of readiness. States and local governments were encouraged to adopt and track the findings and lay the foundations for grade-level reading ability for all children by the end of third grade. Considering the interrelated components of readiness and the importance of multiple preentrance factors, the partners of the Initiative framed the concept with a formula for success. Ready children are prepared by ready families, ready communities, ready services, and ready schools. Thus, the life contexts of the child are fully appreciated, and prior experience is considered fundamental to the child's readiness for learning in the primary grades. Measurable indicators continue to emerge and include factors in such areas as social-emotional, language, and cognitive development.

Citing the importance of early experience and the reciprocal interrelatedness of experience and development, while also addressing the trend toward increasing academic demand and next-grade expectations in the early years, the National Association for the Education of Young Children (NAEYC) drafted a comprehensive position statement on DAP (Bredekamp & Copple, 1997). Familiar core values of the statement champion an appreciation for the uniqueness and value of childhood. The importance of knowledge regarding the learning and development of the child is prioritized. The context of family, culture, and society; the individual nature of each child; and the need for the realization of the child's full potential are recognized. DAPs for the education and well-being of children are designed within a decision-making process that flows from the professional's knowledge of the child based on these principles and from articulated assumptions about learning and child development.

With acceptance of the supposition that the understandings of young children are progressively and actively constructed, expanded, and reorganized through direct experience, constructivism forms one foundation for the educational application of DAP. The value of play is upheld, the need for guided practice (scaffolding) is demonstrated, and the assumption of a variety of learning styles is clear. Developmentally appropriate curriculum offers the right challenge to the actively participating child and deemphasizes teacher-led, whole-group instruction. It serves all areas of development, including cognitive, social, emotional, linguistic, aesthetic, and physical, and builds on the child's own knowledge and ability with integrated content. Developmentally *inappropriate* classrooms, in contrast, have been described as largely offering (in addition to whole-group, teacher-directed methods) isolated instruction with an emphasis on skill development in the cognitive domain and a predominance of abstract pencil-and-paper activities.

Practice within a developmentally appropriate model draws on *both/and* thinking to create a balanced approach and to address criticism surrounding a number of hotly debated issues in education (Bredekamp & Copple, 1997, p. 23). According to NAEYC, for example, children benefit from *both* meaningful experimentation *and* guided instruction from others, *both* predictable structure *and* flexible routine. Further criticism directed toward the appearance of DAP as having more relevance to European American middle-class children has been quieted somewhat by NAEYC's own restatement of its core values and by recent research. Empirical findings from one of a series of studies comparing developmentally appropriate and inappropriate early childhood classrooms (Burts et al., 1993) support the benefits of DAP for children of low socioeconomic status in the United States, regardless of racial background or gender. In other research, commonalities in practice elements are also found in non-Western nations (McMullen et al., 2005). Research continues in an effort to design and test the psychometric properties of a variety of rating tools that measure DAP without sole reliance on teacher self-report. Dialogue is ongoing regarding the identification of DAP, assessment of child outcomes, and the need for flexible adjustment of teaching practices to equitably address the needs of all children.

Once again, teachers and OTs must develop a mutual understanding of terminology and concepts. OTs may hold a different perception of the influence of environment, looking uniquely at room arrangement, materials, the complexity of sound and visual space, as well as routine and pace. Appropriate challenge can be highly individual, and both professionals lend crucial understanding of its application to the education of a given child. DAP is a broad concept, and OTs and teachers have much to share regarding the interplay of all domains of learning.

Laudable efforts to explore and define the concepts of school readiness and DAP are not without significant challenge. In the age of accountability, pre-K curricula are becoming more formalized under pressure from policy makers to have children who are ready make the transition to elementary school (Pianta, 2007). Because the content of the kindergarten curriculum is becoming increasingly academic, 5-year-olds are expected to be ready with more substantial knowledge in measurable skills having a contemporary emphasis on language, literacy, and quantitative concepts (Kagan & Kauerz, 2007). Thus, the "educationalizing" (Kagan & Kauerz, 2007, p. 11) of pre-K programming is narrowing a focus onto the cognitive and academic domains of development and is at variance with the trusted views of the masters of educational theory, who favored a scaffolded learning environment that is individualized to follow the flexible and changing interests of young children as knowledge is constructed.

This trend to facilitate success, achievement, acceleration, and effectiveness creates new tension for teachers and OTs who observe a shift away from movement and play as fertile ground for creative learning experiences toward instructional methodologies that increasingly mirror those offered to older children in school.

THE BRAIN: LAB TO CLASSROOM

Designated the "decade of the brain" (Bush, 1990), the 1990s witnessed a vast and rapid expansion of research on the structure and function of the brain, which was made possible by technologies including computed tomography (CT), positron emission tomography (PET), magnetic resonance imaging (MRI), functional MRI (fMRI), and magnetoencephalography (MEG) (Sousa, 2001). Sophisticated medical instruments remarkably allow the focused x-ray of brain cross-sections, the real-time localized response of the brain to various stimuli, or the activity of the brain as the subject thinks a thought or performs an action. The discoveries of neuroscientists, vital to the care of individuals with specific neurological trauma, have gradually filtered to the field of education and have been translated into *brain-compatible* teaching strategies. Educators often refer to the *science of learning* or the *science of teaching* as an increasing number of resources regarding brain-based learning are offered in the literature in support of constructivist methods.

Scientists have demonstrated the highly interactive nature of the pattern forming, self-organizing brain, which manipulates information in countless ways (Sousa, 2001). Thus, for example, the right-brain, left-brain dialogue has been informed by new understandings; the nature of the limbic system as the seat of emotions has been modernized; and the suggestion of semiautonomous multiple intelligences has been reexamined in light of the remarkably integrative processes of learning, knowing, and doing. Research has discovered the biorhythms of learning and the vital influences of nutrition and rest. It has exposed gender differences and discovered the neurochemical and structural determinants of attention, memory, and transfer. It has ascertained the interactive constituents of learning and emotion. It has elevated music, art, and humor in the process of learning and demonstrated the power of movement in learning and self-regulation. The current literature ranges from a treatise of learning at the micro level of the neuron's synapse (LeDoux, 2002) to a broader application of research in the various works of Jensen (2000a, 2000b, 2004), the National Research Council (2000), Sousa (2001), Wolfe (2001), and Wolfe and Nevills (2004).

Although researchers do caution against the premature or inconsistent application of advancing scientific understanding to daily classroom practice, contemporary teachers may now refer to a menu of working definitions of intelligence. They have at their disposal a burgeoning body of knowledge regarding the brain's ability to process information, the capacity of working memory, as well as the process of long-term memory storage and retention. They can choose from a vast array of published strategies to enhance attention, chunk information for meaning, connect new knowledge to past experience, and generally motivate their students to learn across all subject areas.

DYNAMIC ASSESSMENT
AND DYNAMIC PERFORMANCE ANALYSIS

Based on the works of Lev Vygotsky, dynamic assessment contrasts starkly with traditional standardized psychometric measurement and is finding a place in the professional methodologies of teachers and therapists. The dynamic interaction among student, environment, and task is recognized in the model of cognition itself. Cognition is not seen as fixed and stable, but rather as dynamic in response to changes in activity or context (Toglia, 2005). The child's internal functions of cognition interact with the external environment, the components of the task, and the social relationships from which he or she gleans instructional cues. What the child comfortably accomplishes in the therapy room is often found to be challenging in a more complex or demanding environment where the physical, sensory, and instructional components may tax a fragile problem-solving ability and thwart the automaticity of task performance. Cognition, therefore, is seen as modifiable and sensitive to the characteristics of environment and task (Toglia, 2005).

Traditional standardized testing probes for skills and abilities that the child demonstrates independently and represents the core of completed development at a given point in time (Haywood & Lidz, 2007). During dynamic assessment, guided instruction is offered systematically, with the goal of identifying learning barriers or obstacles and determining the type and intensity of interventions that improve performance. Thus, assessment is contextualized within the ZPD, amplifies a vivid depiction of the child, and is highly supportive of school achievement and occupational performance.

Dynamic assessment answers a very different question when compared with "static" standardized testing. In contrast to a quantitative statement of disability or an identification of the disability and its severity, dynamic assessment probes the possibility of *qualitative change* in performance in response to cues and modifications by looking at whether performance can be changed and what changes it (Toglia, 2005). Thus, the circumstances of *best* performance are understood, and appropriate strategies can be implemented in scaffolding the child's growth. In contrast, variations in traditional standardized test results may be interpreted as errors in the psychometric properties of the test itself. Although useful for diagnostic purposes, conventional assessment does not necessarily inform intervention. As a preventive measure or in conjunction with standardized measurement, dynamic assessment begins an immediate process of strategy trials at the level of core instruction.

Similarly, the OT who observes a child in the natural classroom environment uses dynamic performance analysis (DPA) in analyzing actual performance as the child participates in school-related occupations (Polatajko, Mandich, & Martini, 2000). In doing so, the therapist becomes aware of both internal and external factors that either contribute to or inhibit educational performance. DPA is considered a top-down qualitative assessment approach designed to solve real problems holistically and recognize not only the student–environment–task interplay, but also the possibility of variable paths to successful performance. Conventional task analysis, in contrast, assumes a singular, sequential, and bottom-up approach to activity completion, with the goal of completing the task as it is "normally done." Interventions based on DPA are likely to be a better match to the actual interactive components that influence the unique performance of the child in the natural education environment.

Standardized assessment will not, and should not, lose its place as a crucial portrayal of independent student ability and as a central tool in the identification of need. However, current practices in the public schools, including professional time constraints and a continuing tendency toward pull-out assessment and intervention models, appear to impede the contextualized and dynamic assessment of both the barriers and the constructive influences on learning at all tiers of instruction, as well as the ongoing evaluation of academic and behavioral progress. I believe that this is a direct result of limited pragmatic awareness of the intimate relationship among all domains of learning and of the interactive influence of student, environment, and task. To underscore the partnership of all members of the education team is to adorn collaborations with complete conversation.

POLICY:
IN THE DRIVER'S SEAT

The daily practices of OTs, teachers, and students are framed by state and district policy within the overarching framework of federal law in the form of education acts. Driving documents, such as the No Child Left Behind Act (NCLB) of 2001 (PL 107-110) and IDEA 2004, will undoubtedly continue to evolve and be renamed as successive administrations bring alternative philosophical foundations and new research is accessed.

Since the inception of NCLB in 2001, the Center on Educational Policy (CEP), an independent nonprofit organization, has issued several annual reports offering broad findings regarding the impact of the federal Act and its commanding influence on both teaching and learning. Based on the results of its nationally representative surveys, CEP has found, for example, that the majority of responding school districts has substantially increased elementary instructional time for English language arts (ELA) and/or math in order to emphasize the content of those subjects on state tests used for accountability under the provisions of NCLB (CEP, 2007).

Other findings include efforts by administrators and individual teachers to align district and classroom curricula with state-mandated assessments through such strategies as adopting entirely new ELA and math programs, identifying instructional redundancies and gaps, carefully pacing daily instruction, and matching instruction to published state standards designed to reflect the federal educational priorities. In addition, teaching is described as more prescriptive as teachers and administrators analyze and apply both state test data and local achievement scores to inform and adapt instruction and to design goals for improvement (CEP, 2007). Noting a consequent reduction of instructional time for subjects and areas that are not targeted for federal accountability, such as science, music, art, social studies, recess, and physical education, CEP recommends additional state testing to assess and monitor the progress of other core subjects, including social studies and science.

The burdens of meeting the demands of NCLB, along with challenges of accountability, documented teacher perception of pressure to raise state test scores, and inadequate funding, are cited by CEP as negative effects of the federal Act (CEP, 2006). Positive effects include high expectations for student learning, the increasing alignment of instruction with standards, and the prescriptive use of test data. Among its recommendations, CEP urges attention to a balanced curriculum that offers students a wide offering of core subjects including physical activity and the arts.

Individual states respond to the federal legislation by drafting specific learning requirements for each grade level. In the state of Washington, for example, *Essential Academic Learning Requirements* (EALRs) and *Grade Level*

Expectations (GLEs) are established with the contribution of educators and parents and are published by the Washington Office of Superintendent of Public Instruction (2005). Of particular interest to OTs in Washington schools are the GLEs for writing. The kindergartner, for example, is expected to produce reasonably spaced upper- and lowercase letters, whereas the first grader should place spaces between words and sentences. By second grade, writing is expected to be legible and show consistency of formation, spacing, and size. Writing generation at the kindergarten level calls for the ability to draft simple sentences using some high-frequency spelling words or beginning and ending sounds. The first-grade student writes complete sentences using phonetic spelling with beginning, middle, and ending sounds. The Washington State EALRs reflect a belief in the reading–writing link. Thus, reading programs may require the youngest child to form letters with pencil and paper to facilitate an understanding of the sound–letter correspondence.

CAUTION:
KIDS AND STRESS

The issue of stress in children has increasingly become the subject of research, as well as the anecdotal accounts of education professionals. This author admits to a particular concern for the stress factors influencing young children in school. Stress responses are often exhibited by children who experience conditions for adaptation that are unusually demanding and that excessively expend their energy reserves (Hart et al., 1998). Coping abilities are exceeded in response to a perceived threat to well-being and may result in physical or behavioral responses (Fallin, Wallinga, & Coleman, 2001; Sharrer & Ryan-Wenger, 2002). Children with attention-deficit/hyperactivity disorder (ADHD), learning disability, and speech and language delays, for example, have been identified as exhibiting disproportionate stress behaviors (Arnold et al., 2005; Beitchman, 2005). The school environment itself has been implicated, with school density and class size identified as stress factors. Recently, the microclassroom environment has been examined, including the amount of space per child, with implications for both academic achievement and behavior (Maxwell, 2003). As space per child decreased in the classroom, boys were found to be more vulnerable to behavioral disturbance, whereas girls' achievement scores skewed negatively.

Curriculum, specifically the compression of academic expectations toward the earliest grades, is now a frequent focus of attention. When policy and standards meet DAP and child-centered approaches, stress in young children can be the result. In a 2006 article, "The New First Grade: Too Much Too Soon?" author Peg Tyre addressed the issue of earlier reading expectations and frequent testing for children as young as 6 years. Whereas many children do well under the new standards, failure is the outcome for others, which further creates a deleterious effect on a prized attitude of life-long learning. Remedial instruction is increasingly available, but the pressure on children can be acute, originating from a variety of sources from federal policy to published early learning materials to parent demand. Standards and accountability run headlong into teacher sensitivity to such learning qualities as creativity, natural investigation, diligence, and social-emotional development. As evidence of change in the swing of the pendulum, Tyre reported "dialing back," which includes the banning of standardized testing of young children in Wales and a "slowed-down" approach in some American schools.

Inspired by this widespread concern, Burts and colleagues conducted a series of studies documenting observed stress behavior in young children enrolled in DAP and developmentally *in*appropriate classrooms (Burts, Hart, Charlesworth, & Kirk, 1990; Burts et al., 1992, 1993; Hart et al., 1998). The studies applied the terminology as defined by NAEYC, looking for such practices as the predominance of rote learning; direct discrete skill instruction; highly structured, large-group activity; and excessive abstract pencil and paper tasks as indicators of developmental *in*appropriateness at the kindergarten level. Inappropriate materials included frequently used workbooks and worksheets and standardized testing. Conversely, child-selected activity, center selection, explorative learning, and minimization of whole-group transitions were considered developmentally appropriate for the youngest elementary students.

In these studies, measured stress behaviors were passive or directed toward self, others, or objects. Examples included withdrawal, nail biting or teeth grinding, physical hostility, pencil tapping, or destruction of materials. Summarizing the findings of the early studies, Hart and colleagues (1998) noted that children enrolled in developmentally inappropriate kindergarten classrooms exhibited significantly greater stress levels when compared with their counterparts in DAP classrooms. Economically disadvantaged children and boys were particularly vulnerable to stress when participating in the developmentally inappropriate kindergartens. All children in DAP classrooms, however, regardless of socioeconomic status or gender, exhibited fewer indicators of stress, a finding of support for the equitable benefit of DAP for all children.

Lengthy center activity (in which behavior tends to deteriorate without teacher guidance over time), transitions, and waiting time are particularly problematic with regard to observed stress, even in DAP classrooms. In fact, teacher unavailability was noted more frequently in the more appropriate classrooms in which individual child testing was occurring, thus preventing the ability of the teacher to monitor and guide the group (Burts et al., 1990). Considering the wide chronological and developmental ranges present in most kindergartens, it should be of particular interest to both elementary educators and OTs that kindergarten teachers as far back as the 1980s identified developmentally unmanageable academic tasks as causing the highest incidence of stress symptoms in children, with the severity of symptoms ranking second only to parental separation or divorce (Wiedey & Lichtenstein, 1987). Although mild stress can be motivating for children and not all stress is harmful, the multiple challenges that the young child may experience outside of school can be complicated by developmentally inappropriate practices inside the classroom (Hart et al., 1998).

After nearly 30 years in the public schools, I have become acutely aware of the competing demands weighing on our nation's youngest learners. Kindergarten and first-grade teachers have expressed concern regarding the appropriateness of the curriculum and have described physical indicators of stress in their students. My colleagues and I have been consulted when young children simply refuse to write, and 5- and 6-year-old children are routinely referred to occupational therapy for possible fine motor delay as manifested in early handwriting. Waiting time, implicated in stress research and considered developmentally *in*appropriate, which results in elevated noise making and nonpurposeful or *roaming* behavior is often observed as teachers of young children are compelled to lead isolated reading groups or administer individual achievement tests as early as kindergarten.

The increasing demands for subject coverage have constrained the natural tendency of the young child to lose him- or herself in a favored activity. As I was observing in a kindergarten classroom near the time of this writing, an apologetic young teacher turned to me after ending a brief coloring and drawing session and expressed frustration at having to cut the time short, but, in her words, she could not otherwise "fit everything in." As she instructed the children to put their materials away, one little boy dropped his head and slipped his drawing to the floor. He made the transition to circle time but crossed his arms and disengaged. Unfortunately for teachers and children, inadvertent tension is often created between academic standards and DAP, and a teacher's desire to meet the developmental needs of the children seems to be superseded by the requirements and pace of the curriculum.

FINAL THOUGHTS

The first stages toward a prevention model at all levels of instruction and intervention involve recognition of the mutual influences at work in the educational environment. These include the variations and commonalities of professional theory and educational concept and an awareness of the impact on the content, timing, and pace of curriculum derived from research and policy. Informed collaboration, framed by the balance of student, environment, and task and versed in the knowledge shared broadly across school-based professions creates a much needed monitor on the developmental appropriateness of program, the readiness of children to happily and successfully engage in the activities of school, and the readiness of schools to receive all children.

As a foundation for future collaborations, whether at the level of targeted and intensive interventions or core instruction, the following chapters offer an exploration of mutual understandings of the movement–learning link. They also include the process of knowledge sharing from OT to teacher to investigate fine motor, handwriting, and sensory processing domains as they apply to the K–3 classroom. The student–environment–task interplay is also further examined. Finally, there are practical applications and suggestions offered to utilize student, environment, and task to frame partnerships, plan educational strategies, and problem solve the barriers to learning in a preventive model.

2

Movement, Occupation, and Learning

Virtually every educational activity or learning occupation involves the engagement of the body and the generation of movement. With the simplest task of raising the hand, the child signals attention and understanding. The quietest reader has active eyes and page-turning fingers. The engrossed writer utilizes meticulous, refined, and sequenced movements, the complexity of which is scarcely credited. The young child's body cannot help but disclose the inner life of emotion. Little hands are engaged in nearly every learning task. Simply stated, little bodies are learning partners whose movements and activities are reflected in the brain and whose traces in the world evidence the mind's intent, achieve its purposes, alter its structure, manifest its affect, calm and regulate its attention, and direct its play and work in school.

Movement and learning are linked. Exploring this powerful connection and establishing its foundations will enable its influence to operate for best educational performance and will sustain the art of teaching the moving child.

INVESTIGATING THE MOVEMENT–LEARNING LINK

If learning professionals are going to collaborate to provide the best educational services for children, and if they are going to challenge children while concurrently enabling their ability to be alert, relaxed, focused, and joyful learners, then they should agree on two important points:

1. The student, environment, and task components of occupational performance in the educational environment are not separable.

2. The functions of cognitive, motor, attentional, social-emotional, sensory, and motivational behaviors are not separable.

The movement–learning link represents a natural field study and a lucrative demonstration of the opportunity and need for knowledge sharing across school-based professions. Movement and learning link teachers and occupational therapists (OTs) in the education of young children.

Typically developing 5-year-olds enter kindergarten with a gross motor competency sufficient to navigate them through the various school environments, maintain seated postures with reasonable attention, and stand and walk in a fairly straight line. Inadequate inhibition of motor impulses, however, is the rule rather than the exception and is part of the energy, charm, and challenge of the young child in school. In K–3 classrooms, gathering young children into ordered learning is a fine art, and structure often seems indispensable in maintaining the focus and pace required to meet grade-level expectations (GLE). Movement and attention can seem antithetical. Quiet postures are coaxed into "listening" positions with "criss-cross-apple-sauce" and "hands in lap" directives, and still bodies may be deemed the best indicator of readiness for learning.

Fine motor abilities, teachers often find, can be widely divergent among children and yet heavily underlie the serious academic expectations of today's K–3 curriculum. Given the array of pre-K social and educational experiences available to families today, it is generally anticipated that entering kindergartners will demonstrate a readiness for higher cognitive challenges and literacy foundations. Although this may indeed be the case, little hands are still attached to 5-year-old bodies that are maturing at their own pace and will continue to accrue considerable motor readiness for future complex tasks given unfettered play and practice and motor-based learning activities. Young learners still color, cut, and paste, but are more frequently required to write and spell. We ask a lot of little hands, which might rather follow the larger movements of the whole arm and might struggle to obey the conventions of fine motor specialization.

The theoretical framework for the movement–learning link is not new to educators and OTs. Piaget outlined four stages in the development of intelligence, with the sensorimotor period laying the foundation as infants move and act in the environment (Evans, 1973). They are not passive recipients of experience, but active participants in the dance between nature and nurture. Physical knowledge of concrete objects is mentally transformed into abstraction by way of children's actions as they play with and manipulate the materials in their surroundings.

Maria Montessori decried the contemporary suppression of movement in the educational environment, considering it to be "sadly neglected" and mistakenly regarded as "something less noble than it actually is" (Montessori, 1989, p. 136). Continuity should be evident between body and mind in her educational paradigm, and mental development is considered to be connected with and dependent upon the child's movements.

Personality is expressed through movement, which serves both the intellectual and the social. The child's intelligence is particularly revealed in the work of little hands, which are guided by thought and act in the world. Thus, in the methods of Montessori learning and the manipulation of materials are vitally linked.

A. Jean Ayres (1972), in her groundbreaking work on the relationship between sensory integration and learning disabilities, counted movement as a powerful organizer of sensation for functional use and a mediator of the higher integrative functions of cognition and learning. Through a comparison of available neurological evidence of the brain's ability to integrate sensory information and the observations of children who manifested both learning disability and poorly planned and executed movement patterns, Ayres developed a therapeutic intervention strategy designed to mitigate many of these children's symptoms. In sensory integration therapy, movement is used to elicit an adaptive response from the child, calling simultaneously on the child's motor and cognitive-behavioral processes and elevating the organization of the movement–learning link.

Howard Gardner (1993) broadened the view of cognition and education by describing individual patterns of intelligence in addition to logical-mathematical and linguistic domains, which had long held top priority in the classroom. A child may rely heavily on spatial intelligence in an effort to envision a mental model of his or her environment and to use that model for successful problem solving. The child with superior musical intelligence, for example, appreciates the patterns of music in composition or performance. If a child's bodily kinesthetic intelligence is keen, he or she will learn best through educational activities that engage the body in movement or allow the creation of a product. The theory of a semiautonomous nature and separate memory capacity of each of the intelligences (Gardner, 1999) is a concept that finds variable support in current neuroscience research regarding the interconnectedness of the brain (Sousa, 2001). The theory has, however, awakened the educational community to the existence of diverse entry points to knowledge and a more inclusive conceptualization of the range of human intellectual potential. Attention to the concept of diverse learning styles, or approaches to learning, has been a beneficial outcome of Gardner's treatment of multiple systems of intelligence.

Kieran Egan (1997) described five kinds of understanding, with somatic (bodily) knowledge as the early and primary mediator of meaning that remains fundamental throughout the lifespan. It is the body, in its contact with such attributes as hot/cold and soft/hard that first learns conceptually in a literal dimension and contributes to vivid forms of thought below the level of language. Egan exhorts the preservation of somatic understanding as holding key educational value in the contemporary climate of intellectual and logical-mathematical primacy.

The current emphasis on language and writing as mediators of knowledge reduces the urgency to recruit movement for the child's engagement in the imaginative world of mythical thinking and lore. Mythical understanding, however, is a natural entry point to knowledge for children through age 8 and involves more metaphorical and abstract thinking than once presumed possible by the young learner. In fact, the young child's ability to grasp metaphor is considered to be superior to that of the older child or adult. It is also vital to the construction of knowledge and logic and opens a vast array of imagistic and affectively charged instructional possibilities. In Egan's *An Imaginative Approach to Teaching* (2005), children linger happily in oral language and storytelling, rhyme, rhythm and pattern, mental imagery and humor, mystery, and, of course, play. All are afforded primacy as cognitive tools as weighty as formal literacy training in reading and writing, and all are perfect companions to movement.

CONFIRMATION IN NEUROSCIENCE

Although theoretical support for the movement–learning link is not new, convincing neurophysiological evidence has surfaced more recently. Since the 1970s, our understanding of the integrated nature of brain, body, and mind has increased exponentially with the research of neuroscientists and neurophysiologists, occupational and physical therapists, pediatricians, psychologists, and educators. Current neuroscience investigations depict an elegantly coactive system of dependent or synchronized circuits that are delicately balanced in the active, typically developing child. Where we once referred primarily to observed behavioral indicators of isolated growth in the form of developmental milestone schedules and sequences, we have now begun to assimilate old knowledge with new and recognized that all movement in service to grade-level expectations is intimately connected with learning, thinking, feeling, doing, and attending. Increasingly, published materials directed specifically to teachers highlight the science and neurology of learning in the trend toward brain-based education (Jensen, 2000a, 2004; National Research Council, 2000; Sousa, 2001; Wolfe, 2001; Wolfe & Nevills, 2004).

A past perspective of motor and cognitive functions as discrete and separable may have been a natural sequel to the understanding of underlying brain functions as equally discrete and separable. New perspective reflects an inclusive picture of the integrated nature and efficiency of the brain and the coactivation of multiple levels in all learning. Supplementing the evidence found in brain research and prompting further investigation of the movement–learning link is the increasing awareness of the coexistence of functional cognitive and motor disabilties demonstrated in children with a variety of neurobehavioral disorders.

At the center of the research is the cerebellum, which is a structure the size of a baseball that is tucked behind and under the brain's cerebral cortex and packed with more neurons than the remainder of the nervous system combined (Diamond, 2000) (see Figure 2.1). Once credited solely with the control and timing of movement, balance, and posture, the cerebellum is now confirmed to be coactive in a neural circuit comprised of other motor and sensory centers and with the control center for most complex cognition—the prefrontal cortex. Unquestionably, the cerebellum is active in motor learning, particularly in the early stages of task learning, during novel tasks, and during challenging or changing task demands. As a partner in the neural circuit connected with the prefrontal cortex, the cerebellum is additionally involved in information processing; mental tasks, such as mental arithmetic, mental imagery, and mental word and use association; and sensory perception and function, such as the tactile recognition of geometric shapes. It is also a player in the nonmotor functions of motivation, emotion, and memory storage of behaviors that are learned (Melillo & Leisman, 2004).

Once a skill is fairly established, the participation of the cerebellum decreases, demonstrating its critical role in learning automaticity and the freeing of higher centers for more complex and conscious thought. Before any learning can take place, however, the cerebellum is actively providing a level of baseline arousal, which prepares the brain to process all information (Melillo & Leisman, 2004). It does this in its intimate connection with movement. While the body moves in space, the cerebellum, via its connec-

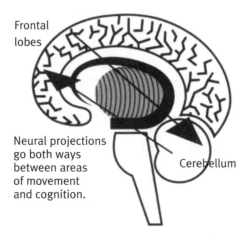

Frontal lobes

Neural projections go both ways between areas of movement and cognition.

Cerebellum

Figure 2.1. The cerebellum in the movement–learning link.

tion to the primary sensory relay structure (the thalamus), receives continuous stimulation from sensory receptors located in the spinal postural muscles and joints. These muscles, which are constantly responding to gravitational forces, provide the only continuous flow of alerting sensation to the brain. Other sensation, including visual or auditory, is more variable and episodic, whereas gravity is a constant. This type of sensory input, which is sent to the brain from receptors in the muscles and joints, is called *proprioception*. It provides the awareness of body position and movement in space and body position and movement in relation to other body parts. Proprioception specifically refers to the body's relationship to gravity. Without the movement of the body, therefore, the cerebellum and its neural circuit would not be effectively stimulated, and the brain would simply not be alert enough to learn. Thus, it is no mystery why we twist, turn, and stretch our spine when we are drowsy or lethargic.

Within a functional framework in studies of the specific relationship to cognition, both working memory and verbal fluency have been found to be related to motor performance in young children (Wassenberg et al., 2005), and the cerebellum is now known to be activated in word generation tasks (Rapoport, van Reekum, & Mayberg, 2000). Language and motor function are further linked in the understanding of spatial concepts (e.g., left-right, up-down), in the vocabulary of time (e.g., fast-slow), and in the ability to both describe and perform movement sequences (e.g., first-then).

Gesture itself is a movement-based language, that is, a link between concept and speech (Armstrong, Stokoe, & Wilcox, 1995). The brain is not "freestanding" in the demonstration of knowledge, but it will use the body to communicate with the simplest flicker of motion or with the complex loops and lines of handwriting. For children who lack linguistic competence, gesture can convey knowledge with greater sophistication than speech and is often generated without conscious awareness (Pine, Lufkin, & Messer, 2004). Children who gesture while talking can sometimes convey an emerging understanding, which belies a clumsy verbal explanation or reflects an idea that is still in formulation. Although counterintuitive, a mismatch between a child's gesture and speech is a sign of knowledge in transition and can convey receptivity to teacher instruction, according to Pine and colleagues. Choice of left or right hand use for gesture-as-language may precede the developmental establishment of hand preference and may be evident in the early manual signs of children with hearing impairments, even before such preference is obvious in object manipulation (Armstrong et al., 1995).

Gesture, however, is more than paralinguistic and is considered integral to thinking itself. Have you ever given driving directions to someone over the phone? Chances are your hands are busy in spatial demonstration, even though your listener does not benefit from the visual aid. Gesture is a reflection of the embodied mind—a physical organizer of thought and sequence of thought—and can be a private motor supplement to the clarity of the mental process. Finally, the ability to use visual-motor skill to demonstrate *procedures* and how-to's is not linguistic at all, rather it represents a form of knowledge sharing that can pass from parent to child, teacher to student, expert to apprentice, and generation to generation.

Because most movement is driven by intent and goal directedness, the motor control system is a working partner with cognition in perfect organization and intricate communication. The system is so elegant that even *imagined* action activates the motor cortex while movement output is withheld (Jeannerod, 2003). In addition, the observation of another's actions will evoke the same neural discharge that occurs when individuals perform the action themselves (Iacoboni, 2003). This ability to mirror action, including the subtleties of facial expression, is critical in human interaction, learning, and empathy. It is considered to be the neural basis of imitation, which is implicated in the study of social thinking or *theory of mind* and the challenges of children with autism.

Implicit learning is centered in the body and occurs outside of conscious awareness (Jensen, 2000b). It is powerfully elicited by movement in skill-based or procedural processes and endures much longer than explicit learning through the memorization of facts and data. The child learns implicitly through experimentation and trial-and-error; the teacher transmits implicit learning through role modeling and demonstration. Among Jensen's ten reasons for offering implicit learning opportunities are the relative ease with which it is imparted, the duration of its effects, its efficiency in freeing higher level thinking, and its integrative linking of body and mind. It is also active in transfer, a dominant principle of learning, that involves the association of new and past understandings and the ability to apply combined learning in the future.

Evidence of the movement–learning link, therefore, implicates the more sedentary lifestyles of children as a major factor in many of the learning differences described by veteran teachers since the 1980s. Reduced attention spans, increasing frustration levels, a decline in verbal abilities, difficulty following the plot lines of reading material, and avoidance of writing have all been reported (Healy, 1990). Inactivity brought on by television viewing and video gaming, along with poor nutrition and the increase in sedentary child care environments has been blamed for an elevated incidence of childhood obesity and changes in learning behavior (Melillo & Leisman, 2004). Considering the intricate neural loop involving cerebellum and higher learning centers, it would seem obvious that no movement is purely motor, and all movement influences baseline arousal and thinking.

The brain shifts attention regularly, and movement provides a natural transition to sustained or renewed focus. Standing alone will increase blood flow and oxygen delivery, increase heart rate by approximately 10 beats per minute, and may increase the speed at which information is processed (Jensen, 2000a). Moving will send about 15% more blood to the brain within 1 minute of rising from a seated position (Sousa, 2001). The subconscious receipt of sensation in the brain arising from the movement of postural muscles is a constant source of brain stimulation and is fuel for learning as surely as oxygen and nutrition.

Research on physical fitness has begun to associate fitness and academic achievement. Using test data compiled by the California Department of Education in 2002, Grissom (2005), matched the results of achievement and fitness testing for students in grades 5, 7, and 9. Higher achievement was associated with higher fitness levels at all three grades, and when mathematics and reading scores were compared, the relationship to fitness was greater for mathematics. Dwyer, Sallis, Blizzard, Lazarus, and Dean (2001) have also documented the contribution of physical fitness to academic performance and further reported on other research findings of positive gains in student attitude, discipline, self-esteem, behavior, and creativity following the initiation of a physical activity program. Although study continues in this area, it would seem that any elimination of fitness activities from the general curriculum would constitute a disservice to the school's overall academic mission, according to Dwyer and colleagues.

FUNCTIONAL IMPLICATIONS

Given current understanding of the theoretical, neurological, and functional connections between movement and learning, we are called to an understanding of the growing child as a dynamic system that is responsive to many forces of change. In the past, the maturational views of some developmental specialists envisioned a child primarily driven by genetics and awaiting brain development as nature's singular incentive. More recently, dynamic systems theory inspired a new synthesis of motor development as the interplay of neural and biomechanical properties of the body, the constraints and supports of the environment, and the potentially changing requirements of the task (Thelan, 1995). The efficient pattern of walking, for example, is a self-organized solution that is a product of human motor system properties in concert with the environmental influences of ground and gravity. These constants make walking the natural choice for everyday locomotion, whereas hopping or jumping are eliminated as less tenable options. As Thelan interestingly reveals, hopping, as seen with astronauts, appears to be the more efficient choice on the moon where gravity exerts an entirely different influence. Teachers should be grateful for the stronger gravitational forces governing children here on earth!

In Thelan's (1995) model, task is the "driving force for change" (p. 86) because experience causes the brain to mature just as maturation of the brain enables new experience to unfold. Cognition and movement, with regard to the movement–learning link, emerge from the same dynamic interplay of child, environment, and task. In fact, a definition of the young child's brain as *plastic* means that it is modifiable in response to both activity and experience (Melillo & Leisman, 2004). Motor learning theory continues to evolve, with new appreciation for the brain's ability to select from a group of neural connections in order to match and refine motor activity given the conditions of the environment. Whatever the specific theoretical framework, however, there is broad acceptance for the interaction of systems in the production of movement, which lends support for the need to consider the student factors, environmental components, and task demands in all areas of occupational performance, including education.

It would seem, therefore, nearly impossible to evaluate the child's "real" abilities in the absence of simultaneous assessment of all components of occupational performance in context. This is an important point educationally, as the student can either succeed or fail, self-organize or become overwhelmed by the combined demands of academic expectation in the classroom. *Functional ability*, a term frequently used by OTs, acknowledges this interconnection and refers to the child's ability to complete a task in its natural context. Functional ability is not consistent, but changes with the variation of task and environmental demands. In motor terms, for example, running on a smooth surface may be well within the child's capability, whereas moving on uneven ground is a challenge. The ability to run is an inherent characteristic of the child, but the features of the environment influence the functional outcome (which is actually true for all of us). Walking slowly is a very different task than moving quickly. Running in a straight line is different from running an obstacle course, which recruits more heavily from other learning domains, such as executive functions for planning, organizing, and self-monitoring, and requires a perceptual overlay in analyzing the quickly changing relationship between self and environment. The nature and demands of task constrain movement. Movement and learning are partners in functional performance.

On a cautionary note, because the modifiability of brain function or plasticity holds that experience is a powerful influence, designed experiences for children can facilitate successful task completion or complicate educational demand beyond a child's best occupational performance. Educational tasks require a variety of movement demands. The learner's ability to understand the nature of the task is certainly foremost as frustration or failure is ensured without it, regardless of motor ability. Movement itself, however, provides a layer of engagement that occurs easily and subconsciously or with difficulty and active concentration. For example, picking up a pencil is a simple task that employs undemanding movement with an observable beginning and end point. Using the pencil to scribble requires a more complex synergy of motion in the hand with a minimal planning component. Using the pencil to write a sentence blends neurodevelopmental and language components, which increases the complexity of the task considerably and integrates several domains of learning. Without a model for the design, evaluation, and modification of task demand, poor functional outcome may be attributed to inherent attributes of the child, ignore the other elements of occupational performance, and set in motion strategies of repeated instruction or tutoring that will only frustrate the child's ability to succeed.

When movement becomes automatic, cognition is freed for higher level functions. However, when at the novice stage, the child's movement usurps conscious attention and draws cognitive resources away from more complex learning. If you don't play tennis, rollerblade, or produce calligraphy, try learning how to do these tasks and you will relate. Parents of toddlers readily share anecdotes of the reduction of babbling when children take their first steps. Physical education teachers and coaches know the value of practice drills to increase movement automaticity and free higher level thinking for tactics and strategies in games and sports.

Three critical factors affect movement automaticity (speed–accuracy interplay) and influence the development of educational and occupational performance. First is an instructional methodology that is appropriate to the child's development and utilizes the child's most efficient and rehearsed motor patterns. For the younger learner, whole-body or whole-arm movements are effectively recruited in the learning of patterns that will have a later, more refined application. Thus, many of the patterns of handwriting are often demonstrated with "air-writing" or "letter postures."

The second factor is the degree to which *unencumbered* practice is allowed. Unencumbered practice is *not* unguided or unsupervised practice; rather, it is the opportunity to rehearse the motor elements of a task in diverse ways *before* additional complex academic components are introduced or layered on. We do not expect children to shout out math facts while they are learning to ride a bicycle. Instead, we allow them time and freedom to exclusively practice the motor challenge for their own safety and success. Should we, then, expect young students to compose a sentence before they have learned and rehearsed the formation of the letters of the alphabet? During practice, the child is free to experiment with various strategies and is more concerned with process than outcome. Developing executive functions are devoted to self-regulation and monitoring within a singular expectation. The child incorporates effective patterns or abandons ineffective patterns and, therefore, improves efficiency. The abandonment of immature strategies favors automaticity. This is reflected in Sousa's counsel that "practice does not make perfect. Practice makes permanent" (2001, p. 99).

The third critical factor affecting movement automaticity and influencing the development of educational and occupational performance is the timing of outcome expectation. Quickly placing a higher academic expectation on a novel motor task may inhibit the experimental stage in the interest of product and outcome and can trap the learning child in a less effective motor stage. In my experience, pencil grasp and printing legibility are often casualties of the early application of handwriting demand.

Does this sound contradictory? Have I not been making a case for the movement–learning link? Have I not acknowledged the effectiveness of constructivist methods that associate old learning with new? It's a matter of timing. Allow foundations to develop automaticity, essentially to become old learning, and their association with new knowledge will happen freely and naturally without frustration or work. This incites many questions regarding the presentation of contemporary literacy programs that are addressed in Chapter 4 of this volume.

MUSIC AND RHYTHM:
MOVEMENT PARTNERS IN LEARNING

Nothing charms movement out of the body more readily than music and rhythm. Music has been linked to blood pressure and pulse rates, muscle activity, and the strengthening of cortical neuron connections (Baumgartner, Willi, and Jäncke, 2007; Chafin, Roy, Gerin, & Christenfeld, 2004; Evers, Dannert, Rödding, Rötter, & Ringelstein, 1999). It engages both hemispheres of the brain by requiring the recognition of patterns, as well as changes in pitch and pace (Jensen, 2000a). Listening to music or embedding information in music has been found to influence memory recall and visual imagery (Sousa, 2001). It extends the working memory capacity of the young child by linking many more bits of information than the child might otherwise recall. Furthermore, adding movement appears to increase the power of the music-rhythm benefit. Creating music, for example, rather than simply listening to it, has been linked to educational advantage. In one California study, piano keyboarding was added as an instructional supplement for preschoolers and resulted in improved spatial-temporal reasoning, whereas computer keyboarding (similar movements without music) did not (Sousa, 2001). Perception of space and spatial attributes of objects is more than visual. Our bodies move in the environment and act on its elements, providing a rich store of information to our understanding. As a child's fingers simultaneously and sequentially land on piano keys, the brain is informed of patterns in space and time and combines the auditory and visual patterns of melody and sheet music.

In another study (Wolfe, 2001), the combination of piano instruction and academics resulted in higher math scores (proportional math and fractions) for inner city second graders, which is not surprising considering the predictable patterning of both math and music. Music can enhance emotional arousal or calm through beat-per-second rhythms. In addition, it is used in the behavioral regulation of children with sensory processing disorders. Rhythm without music is especially fun for children who can create it by tapping, clapping, stomping, marching, and myriad other ways.

WHY WE LET THEM PLAY

It hardly seems necessary to mention the value of play to teachers of 5- to 8-year-old children. After all, the United Nations, at its 1989 Convention on the Rights of the Child, swiftly and widely advanced a legally binding international human rights treaty that specifically addresses play as the right of every child (Office of the High Commissioner for Human Rights, United Nations, 1989). It is unfortunate, however, that play has become a casualty of many factors, including the more rigorous educational standards of the K–3 curriculum. Since the 1980s, children have lost, overall, 12 hours of free time per week (Elkind, 2007), and recess has been eliminated in 40% of American schools (Hirsh-Pasek & Golinkoff, 2003). Most likely, if you teach young children, you are quite aware of the benefits of play and its association with learning, and you lament the inevitability of an increased pace in the classroom and the elimination of blocks of imaginative playtime. Here, we review the link between play and learning and underscore the importance of restoring our wonderment of the rewards of play and the mythical, fantasy-wrapped, imagination-friendly world of childhood, even in school.

Play is a ubiquitous occupation of childhood, and there is no end to the documentation of its nature and benefit. It is described as promoting problem solving and creativity; facilitating motor, language, and literacy development; and encouraging social connectedness (Baumer, Ferholt, & Lecusay, 2005; Bergen, 2002; Bredekamp, 2004; Coolahan, Fantuzzo, Mendez, & McDermott, 2000). Play maximizes concentration and attention, and it engages the child in goal setting, rule following, and turn taking. It is a portal to analytical thinking, which is the foundation of math and science. Play can facilitate convergent or divergent thinking, depending on the nature of the play materials. Convergent materials lead the child to a single, correct solution, as do many of the educational toys on the market today. Divergent materials (e.g., dress-up clothing, traditional blocks) present open possibility and encourage multiple solutions.

Play helps the child to blend the known and the new, to stretch the real into the possible, and to work through the emotions of both. In play, the differences among children, which we might vigilantly document elsewhere, are insulated from interpretation and measurement. There is a freedom in play that is inherently pleasurable, which is reflected in the four critical components of play as defined in Liebschner's work (1992). First, play is free from the external demands of imposed purpose or consequence and from the internal demands of the self. Second, it is bound by some organization and rules, but fluid enough to allow for the ingress and regress of players. Third, repetition of the familiar, although common in play, is not sufficient to keep it alive. Low-level tension thus exists between freedom and rule, known and unknown, familiar and new, real and make believe, and predictable and unpredictable. Without it, or with the excess of tension, play will cease. Fourth, there is no drive in the child to eliminate play, but rather a desire for the continuation of the process, and there is no compulsion toward an end product, even though one may result.

Play is utterly self-satisfying and may abruptly end when the child is satiated. It represents a *self-selected curriculum* (Jenkinson, 2001, p. 5) that can meet or exceed the GLEs of published standards and allows the child nutritive *wallowing time* (p. 30). Play is a priceless educational investment. Unlike interaction with electronic media, natural play launches the child into sensory encounters that shape perceptions of all kinds. In *The Power of Play*, Elkind (2007) recounts three misunderstandings of how young children learn and their relationship to play. First, although children imitate many actions during modeled instruction, they require more nonimposed, self-directed activity than we might allow if we fail to trust their own priorities in play. Second, the perception of young children as *little sponges* (Elkind, 2007, p. 95) assumes their ability to absorb formal instruction at earlier ages, when, in fact, they require time to process and assimilate new information and experience. Third, children learn naturally through self-directed play and may not be ready to find meaning in instruction, even if we urge them to persist.

Play finds a natural place in constructivist methodologies that value child-centered learning, personal meaning building, active construction of understanding, and authentic exploration. Since the late 1990s, investigators have drawn attention to its contributory role in emergent literacy, and play is now at the center of one of the most exhaustive areas of research in the field of early literacy development (Feldman, 2005; Morrow & Schickedanz, 2006; Roskos & Christie, 2001). Oral language; print awareness; phonological awareness as explored in playful word use; ZPD; and children's *appropriation* of knowledge from social encounters, along with the use of symbol, are included as some of the topics of study.

The nature of play as fluid, flexible, and original promotes learning in a way that is quite different from adult-structured, cognitive, and linear instruction. Play is not equivalent to center time, which is more likely to draw the child toward specific learning objectives. It is, in fact, so valued by the child that it has become my personal practice to avoid at all costs scheduling individual therapy sessions during genuine playtime, whether in the classroom or on the playground. In addition to my own aversion to the intentional elimination of an opportunity for play and movement, at no other time have I encountered the tears and sadness that can accompany a disruption of play. It is simply not worth it.

RECESS: IS IT STILL THERE?

Both body and brain are refreshed during recess, and the child is better prepared for the next round of academics. When children struggle with attentional or sensory processing disability, I recommend that the teacher take a close look at the daily schedule. Subjects that require heavy concentration, such as math or science, should be strategically positioned immediately following a recess or physical education class. I will also advocate strongly for every child's right to recess and underscore the inadvertent but counterproductive policy of holding children inside as a consequence of uncompleted work. Whereas the typically performing student may not suffer from the occasional loss of a play or movement break, the elimination of this critical restoration time is a double-edge sword for the child who is struggling academically. When a child who cannot complete or concentrate on the academic classwork is then asked to work longer than his or her peers, he or she is also asked to work for longer periods without the benefit of movement. An unintended outcome is that learning readiness (the child is alert, relaxed, and focused) can decline for subsequent tasks, and both student and teacher may bear the unwelcome consequences.

Instead of eliminating the recess break, teachers often support student productivity with strategies such as eliminating distractions in the classroom environment, setting learning to music, drama, or play, allowing preferential seating near the teacher, modifying the length or demand of the task, providing an individual study carrel, supporting organizational and time management skills, and of course, encouraging implicit learning by embedding movement into everyday instruction.

Recess is losing out to academic coverage all over the country and has actually been eliminated from many school agendas altogether. Counter to expectations, however, test scores have not proven to increase as a result, and excessive instructional phases can actually inhibit learning and retention (Zygmunt-Fillwalk & Bilello, 2005). Even when recess is preserved, many opportunities for powerful and organizing movement sensation that were previously delivered by swings, teeter-totters, and merry-go-rounds have been lost for reasons of safety and liability. Nonetheless, the recuperative value of this brief but essential break from the work of the classroom is advantageous to the self-regulation, social-emotional adjustment, and cognitive efficiency of young students in school. Thankfully, advocacy groups, including children's organizations, teachers, parents, and physicians have rallied to the reclamation of recess, and position statements are available from the National Association for Sport & Physical Education (NASPE), the

National Association of Early Childhood Specialists in State Departments of Education (NAECS/SDE), the National Association for the Education of Young Children (NAEYC), and the Association for Childhood Education International (ACEI) (Zygmunt-Fillwalk & Bilello, 2005).

BOYS IN THE LINK

With little boys once making up as much as 100% of those children referred to me for special education evaluation at the elementary level, I have reason for concern. I began to question the likelihood that student factors, including the ability to attend and self-regulate and the capacity to produce refined (written) work, were compromised by the overly constraining elements of the environment and the excessive and mismatched demands of educational task. I have noted that teachers, too, are becoming increasingly alarmed at the prevalence of behavioral and performance issues for boys in earlier grades. It should be a priority for education team members and policy makers to continue to critically explore the research-based evidence regarding the dynamics and influences of gender as they affect little boys (and girls) in school, particularly as GLEs and curriculum methodologies favor earlier entry into the writing activities of literacy instruction.

Although many behavioral variations are induced by culture and lifestyle, there is significant evidence that is corroborated multiculturally that gender-based learning distinctions reflect biological differences in the organization of the brain (Gurian, 2001; Healy, 2004; Jensen, 2000a, 2000b; Sousa, 2001). Although individual uniqueness across genders is certain and absolutes are not claimed, little boys tend to be louder and more aggressive, impulsive, and active than girls, making the greater outdoors an important regulator of their attention and learning-readiness inside the classroom.

By toddlerhood, little girls tend to outpace boys in the acquisition of verbal ability and hold their advantage through the primary grades (Tyre, 2008). In contrast to the verbal problem-solving strategies of girls, boys rely more heavily on visual-spatial strategies and exploration through gross motor activity and touch. The superior spatial aptitudes of boys may offer the advantage in mental manipulation of the abstract and in deductive exercises. Little girl classmates, however, will tend to have superior language, inductive, and fine motor ability, possibly placing male peers at a disadvantage in managing the language load of the early literacy content and the earlier and more pressing fine motor demands of handwriting. Although lingering cultural preferences may expect emotional competence from him, the little boy can take much longer to process emotional information; have fewer language resources in managing it; and consequently be more distracted after events that upset, worry, or alarm him (Gurian & Stevens, 2005).

The young boy shows a quicker response to the attention demands of the environment, and he is not the better listener. Thus, he may be less receptive to verbal detail and may become more restless during lengthy instructional sessions. He is chemically and metabolically (and anecdotally) driven toward fidgety behavior. Consequently, he is more likely to lose recess time as a consequence of challenging behavior, although he needs the change of pace to feed his body's craving for motion. He may be drawn to the frenetic and spatial allure of visual technology, but his quiet body may object with bursts of overactivity, making it difficult for him to prepare for and transition to the next educational task. Newer, more interactive technologies can be a better match for him educationally. Active learning in the form of object manipulation will not offer the intensity of whole body engagement in the movement–learning link.

Curriculum is not intentionally designed to be preferential, but somehow the needs of little boys may not be satisfied in the current educational paradigm. Statistics are sobering. Although the prevalence of learning disabilities may be fairly equal among boys and girls, boys are *diagnosed* as much as four times more often (Turkington & Harris, 2006). Attention problems are diagnosed, and medications prescribed, more frequently for affluent white males who may encounter intense expectations for academic achievement, and poor African American boys whose schools may be overcrowded and underfunded (Tyre, 2008). Boys are at the center of 80% of school discipline problems, make up 80% of children diagnosed with behavioral disorders, and receive the majority of failing grades (Gurian & Stevens, 2005).

In my experiences and observations, I have seen that boys appear to be struggling in greater numbers. Something is not working as well for them, and many experts implicate an early developmental disadvantage in school. I would add to that the increasing task demands in the multiple and complex environments of school itself, with the trend toward longer periods of quiet or seated work and stationary bodies, even for our youngest learners. With a greater understanding of unique gender differences and with resolution of any lingering sensitivity to the issue, the elements of occupational performance in the classroom can comprehensively address the needs of all students at the level of core instruction. Our mutual goal is to prevent the need for intervention. My hope is that we identify fewer children for specially designed instruction and that my concern for the successful educational performance of little boys is unwarranted.

MOVEMENT AND THE CLASSROOM ENVIRONMENT

I once advised a kindergarten teacher to remove her classroom's chairs and tables until January. I was only half kidding. Without attachment to a chair, and even sometimes with, little bodies are in perpetual flux. Postural movement is in constant response to gravity, and it is the only continuous source of alerting proprioceptive stimulation to the brain. Without it, baseline arousal is not maintained, and young children may drift in one of two directions. Either they become lethargic and inattentive or they burst into motion in a subconscious attempt to regain or maintain learning readiness. A gradual drift will be noticed by the alert adult who can then incorporate remedial strategies. Integrated or embedded movement, however, is both preventive and learner friendly.

This does not mean that the classroom becomes chaotic and noisy. With chairs aside, children's natural postural adjustments on the floor will benefit them in many ways. Tactile opportunities abound as the body contacts the carpet. The abdominal core is strengthened during variable positions and movement transitions. Providing children with clipboards encourages them to lie on their bellies, increasing proximal joint stability in the shoulders and placing the head in an antigravity position. The *holding* and *working* sides of the body are more pronounced when children are coloring or drawing on their bellies, and hand preference may be more obvious and consistent. Placing a large strip of newsprint on the floor creates an opportunity for peer collaboration in the creation of a pictorial masterpiece. The child's visual relationship to the environment changes with the movement of the body and head, and spatial information is gained. Social or group engagement is encouraged in multiple directions.

Without traditional chairs, other options are created. For example, rocking chairs, gliders, therapy balls, T-stools, and bolsters entice movement and rhythm and capture attentional resources. Many teachers have replaced chairs with therapy balls. As a result, they have observed decreased restlessness, increased attending behavior, and extended duration of the limits of concentrated work. One of my friends and colleagues recruits parents to construct T-stools for her kindergartners, and they have now become a standard seating supplement in her classroom. The value of dynamic seating is confirmed in research. Disc cushions on chairs and therapy balls as chair alternatives have both resulted in significant gains in attention and occupational performance in children with attention deficits (Pfeiffer, Henry, Miller, & Witherell, 2008; Schilling, Washington, Billingsley, & Deitz, 2003).

Simply standing can offer more intense thinking stimulation than the seated position. I often recommend allowing a student to work for a while at a higher classroom counter, thus enabling more frequent postural adjustment, arm and shoulder stability while leaning, and proprioceptive stimulation through the antigravity challenge. Taping a long strip of newsprint to the wall creates a *graffiti* center that not only incorporates standing, but also provides a vertical drawing surface that simultaneously brings wrists and fingers into a more mature prehension for crayons and markers.

All materials do not have to be at optimal height for accessibility. Encouraging some reaching and stooping to recover belongings requires

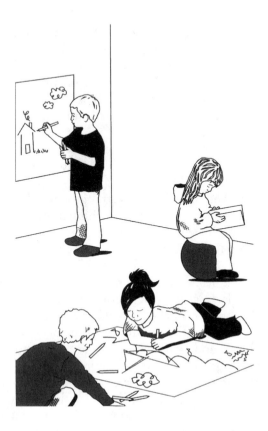

heavy work for muscles and joints, thus providing sensory-loaded movement that regulates learning readiness. Reading nooks can even be located in a loft with a safe ladder to encouraging climbing opportunities not otherwise available. I have seen this in action to the delight of the children.

Once chairs and tables return to the classroom (in January—again, only half kidding), careful attention should be paid to ergonomics and space issues. Every child deserves a good fit in his or her chair, and teachers may need to swap styles to accommodate a variety of body sizes. The 5- to 8-year-old child is growing rapidly, which makes routine visual rechecks of the seating necessary throughout the year. Backs should be supported with pillows for the smaller child. Children's feet should reach the floor and rest comfortably without requiring thighs to hang heavily over the front of the chair. If little legs are constantly swinging or wrapping around chair legs, or if children are always sitting on their heels, then it's time to check chair height or provide a wooden foot support. Taller children may become equally ill at ease in a chair, tucking their legs under the seat and towering above the table.

If feet constantly swing, tuck, or wrap, posture is missing a key component of stability for refined dexterity work. When children are continuously and subconsciously fighting for postural control, attentional resources may be distributed inefficiently and concentration can suffer. The simple recommendation for ergonomic modification once reduced distractibility significantly for one of my second graders who was of short stature. He became much less fidgety, and his sustained concentration improved considerably. The implications for learning were dramatic with just a few adjustments to his seating.

I find that table or desk height can sometimes be a sensitive issue for teachers. As they seek natural student groupings based on constructivist educational theory, desks are brought into contact in groups of two, four, or six. Shared materials are best positioned on same-height tables, regardless of student size. In this case, I try to accommodate the teacher's concerns with primary adjustment to chair size and height and the use of foot rests. In the end, however, every child's postural stability must be given due consideration. Optimal table height can be determined by having students dangle their arms at their side. Elbows should be about 2 inches above the height of the table or desk. When a child is working, the surface will support upright posture while still maintaining a functional distance from paper to eyes.

Adults should be observant of the students' management of space when several children are seated at the same table or desk grouping. Boys tend to require more learning space and may spread materials more widely on the

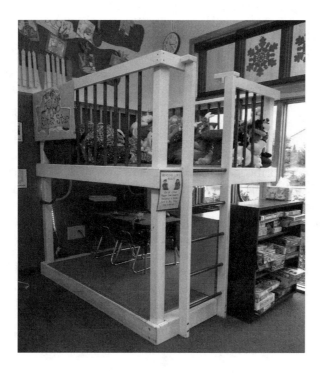

table surface. Close physical proximity may inhibit natural movement and may actually be intolerable to the child with sensory sensitivity or behavioral issues. The relationship between classroom spatial density and stress, according to Maxwell (2003), is instructive regarding the need for optimal space for children. Less space has been associated with a decline in interaction among preschoolers, more solitary play, and less gross motor play. Increased aggression and distractibility have accompanied a decline in square footage for young children in the classroom. Maxwell further found that classroom density negatively influenced girls' reading scores and boys' behavior.

NEUROBEHAVIORAL DISORDERS AND THE MOVEMENT–LEARNING LINK

An investigation of the movement–learning link reveals unquestionable implications for the typically developing child in school. The connection, however, becomes uniquely evident when serving the needs of children with developmental delays.

Just as movement and learning and cerebellum and cerebral cortex were functionally separated in the past, special educators and neuroscientists once viewed common neurobehavioral disorders as discrete disabilities. Melillo and Leisman (2004) suggest, however, that attention deficit disorder (ADD), attention-deficit/hyperactivity disorder (ADHD), learning disability (LD), pervasive developmental disorder (PDD), autism, Asperger syndrome, obsessive-compulsive disorder (OCD), Tourette syndrome (TS), and childhood schizophrenias reflect a continuum of disorders manifesting neurologically as different combinations, asymmetries, and severities of a common underlying neural mechanism. The various combinations of disability along this continuum result in the diverse learning and behavioral symptoms of these disorders. This mechanism is the same neural circuit underlying the movement–learning link!

The high co-incidence of symptoms, including inefficient executive functions of monitoring, self-regulation, and attention; emotional liability; impulsivity; learning and language difficulties; social affiliation challenges; and gross motor and fine motor delays is striking in the functional manifestations of children with diagnosed neurobehavioral disorders. Additional factors, including imbalances of regulating neurotransmitters and hormones, that favor asymmetrical distribution in left or right brain hemispheres can also be evident. Normal functions can be disrupted in any combination and are evident in higher level cortical areas, subcortical areas, natural asymmetries of effective brain function, and size deficiencies of critical brain structures, particularly the cerebellum. Dysfunction can lead to the overactivity or underactivity of structures, which results in the variations of arousal, behavioral, and learning symptoms.

Motor delay is reported in 50%–90% of children with developmental language disorders. Slow early motor milestones and poor vocabulary are associated in children with a familial risk of dyslexia (Viholainen et al., 2006). Motor deficits in imitation, balance, coordination, speech articulation, and hypotonia (low muscle tone) are commonly reported to be present in children with autism, although they may be considered an area of strength relative to more obvious social and communication delays. Melillo and Leisman (2004) describe additional findings of overlapping symptoms, including hyperactive behaviors in children with either ADHD or Tourette syndrome, dopamine deficiencies in children with ADHD or schizophrenia, depressive behaviors in children with Asperger syndrome or OCD, sensory sensitivity and auditory processing delays in children with learning disability or autism. Ineffective global arousal states are common in children with learning disability or ADHD. Delayed hand preference, low muscle tone, poor motor coordination, and attentional difficulties are commonly reported in many of the neurobehavior disorders. Anatomically, the cerebellum has been found to be of smaller size in children with autism, ADHD, and schizophrenia. Multiple disorders are sometimes diagnosed in the same child.

OTs and teachers are faced with these overlapping symptoms in many of the children with whom they work daily. OTs utilize movement as an ally to occupational performance and frequently recommend movement strategies to bind the elements of task demand for struggling learners. Letter formation may be introduced with whole arm motion and multisensory activities. Self-regulation and attending is enhanced with heavy work or resistive movement that increases the intensity of organizing proprioceptive feedback from muscles and joints. Academic tasks, such as spelling or the memorization of math facts, can be paired with rhythmic movement on a therapy ball. Suspended equipment, including platform or bolster swings, are considered indispensable in feeding the movement–learning neural circuit for children with autism or sensory processing disorder. By using movement strategically, the stressed or overwhelmed child is calmed, the lethargic child is alerted, and learning readiness is stabilized. Riding a tricycle, climbing on playground equipment, or playing with a ball can be gateways to planning, organization, sequencing, and attending ability. The options are limitless.

A common thread is becoming increasingly clear. The movement–learning link as regulated by cerebellum and prefrontal cortex, along with other sensory and motor centers in the same neural loop, is not only central to an understanding of the common neurobehavioral disorders of childhood, it is critical to the effective delivery of curricular activities that account for the student–environment–task elements of occupational performance in school. Although some dysfunction can be lifelong, the changes in brain function that result from sedentary lifestyle and the stillness of little bodies in the classroom are correctible, according to Melillo and Leisman (2004).

Developmental coordination disorder (DCD) is a relatively recent diagnostic category that is beginning to replace terminology such as clumsy child syndrome, minimal brain dysfunction, developmental dyspraxia, or perceptual motor difficulty (Barnhart, Davenport, Epps, & Nordquist, 2003; Hadders-Algra, 2002). Considered a chronic and typically permanent condition, DCD is estimated to occur in approximately 5%–8% of all school-age children. Children with DCD experience motor impairment, without evidence of pervasive developmental disorder (PDD) or identifiable neuropathology (e.g., cerebral palsy), that interferes with completion of daily living activities or with achievement in academics. Late achievement of motor milestones, poor athletic performance, and poor handwriting are common functional challenges. The child with DCD may have difficulty choosing the optimal motor strategy and may fail to adjust unsuccessful strategies when attempting to complete a task (Missiuna, Mandich, Polatajko, & Malloy-Miller, 2001).

Children with DCD are heterogeneous as a group, but are often co-diagnosed with language disorder or ADHD and can have empathy disorders common to children with autism (Piek & Dyck, 2004). These comorbidities are frequently assumed to represent discrete phenomena; however, the existence of a common neural circuit in many neurobehavioral disorders of childhood, as described by Melillo and Leisman (2004) and others, inspires important research into underlying causes of these conditions as a group. According to Piek and Dyck (2004), the distinguishing characteristic of children with DCD, although not necessarily causal, is poor visual-spatial processing. Verbal and cognitive-behavioral interventions are showing promise for children with DCD (Missiuna et al., 2001).

☀ The Observations of an Occupational Therapist ☀

Jonathan was a bright kindergartner, perfectly capable of managing the instructional rigors of an all-day blended K–1 classroom—or so his parents and teacher thought. In September, he was a happy, engaged, and productive learner. Certainly, he was energetic, more so than many of his older classmates, but that was to be expected, considering the chronological range of the group. Initially, he followed directions readily and completed his work on time. As the year progressed, however, Jonathan became increasingly wiggly. He was often off topic, and he fiddled relentlessly with materials or left his seat altogether. His attending behavior deteriorated so thoroughly that, when given an opportunity to be the leader of the day, he was unable to convey instructions for the most familiar of classroom activities. His attempt to direct the class in a predictable and routine sequence of tasks required multiple reminders from a very patient teacher. By January, Jonathan required an adult aide to keep him constructively engaged.

It seemed inevitable that Jonathan would be referred for special education evaluation. I was asked to join the team to help determine the reason for his low fine motor productivity. I was also asked to assess his sensory processing abilities, which were suspected in his poor attending and overactive behavior. As is my usual practice, I scheduled a classroom visit and observed Jonathan in his natural surroundings for nearly 2 hours. I happened to be in the classroom on an atypical day, which I initially considered to be an unfortunate circumstance because I wished to see his "typical" behavior. As it turned out, however, the alternative activities of this day proved to be most revealing and informative of this young boy's needs.

During the first part of my observation, with Jonathan at his desk and the remainder of the class quietly engaged in a writing task, Jonathan found everything to do but write. He required numerous reminders to work with pencils, rather than markers. He did not use either as assigned, however, and they were variously tapped, spun, or clicked in and out of their lids. He stood at his desk, leaving his chair unoccupied, and, providing himself with a convenient head start, he wandered the room and chatted with his neighbors.

Relief was soon to come. Because the class had been maintaining a steady and vigorous pace and was slightly ahead of the curriculum schedule, the children were afforded the unusual luxury of constructing a supplemental learning activity. After reading several fairy tales, they were planning, on this day, to act out a familiar story in groups of five. I watched as Jonathan's troupe separated into a corner of the room and assigned to themselves character roles. A first-grade boy appeared to take the natural lead as director and narrator. Jonathan was ecstatic with his assignment as the mean old wolf in the "Three Little Pigs." As they rehearsed, I watched as Jonathan was reprimanded for wielding his props as weapons and for slowing the progress of his supporting cast of pigs. Then, as time went on, something interesting began to happen. Jonathan began to settle down. To my surprise, he learned his lines easily and never once failed to respond to his stage cues. Although still requiring a little extra attention, Jonathan was the meanest, gruffest, most expressive and focused wolf of the day, huffing and puffing with flair and earning a well-deserved round of praise and applause! The ear-to-ear grin was testament to his great satisfaction and pride.

As I left the room, Jonathan's teacher was obviously pleased with his participation that day, and I recall affirming that this active learning method appeared to be just what he needed. The evaluation proved to be negative for developmental delay in any area with the exception of lingering social challenges, and Jonathan was recommended for specially designed instruction only in that domain. Strategically designed active participation was exactly what suited his age, temperament, and sensorimotor needs. The more sedate K–1 blend, with long periods of desk work and quiet concentration that were apparently thought to be a good match for his intellect, proved to restrain his body and impede his readiness to learn cumulatively over time. Needless to say, the evaluation team was wholly supportive of his parents' decision to enroll him in an alternative placement for first grade, one that held the promise of a close movement–learning link. The following fall, I was thrilled to hear of Jonathan's eager participation and productivity in his new environment. He is now doing very well.

As I participate in the activities of K–3 classrooms, I detect a declining incorporation of movement and a dissolving of the partnership between body and cognition. Certainly movement has not been eliminated, and teachers are skilled in designing active strategies and using movement games to maintain motivation and attention. However, I typically note that the priority of math and literacy instruction seems to preclude the engagement of little bodies. Yet, it does not have to be so. Movement activity is more than transitional or a break to get blood flowing again. Movement is not a simple hearkening to the call for developmentally appropriate practice (DAP); it is recruited to aid the child's understanding in a way that linguistic concepts cannot. It accentuates procedures that have more abstract application. It visibly reveals the understanding of the learner and provides ample opportunity for scaffolding. It feeds the learning brain and awakens arousal and enhances learning readiness. Movement draws out the emotions and enhances a memory of the learned event. It is no mystery that our most vivid childhood memories are those that are rich with sensation from the body—a trip to the beach, with the water, salty air, and labored runs through the warm, soft sand; the neighborhood games of kick-the-can late into the summer evening; rides on the biggest, fastest roller coaster in the world; or a frolicking jump in the leaves, or the hay, or the mud.

More and more, active seems to refer to the use of refined manipulatives, which engage only a small part of the child. More instruction is conducted with the aid of the whiteboard and other technologies, which place the child firmly on the floor or in a chair. When teachers read aloud, they use body, gestures, and facial expressions to impart meaning, humor, surprise, and suspense. Yet, listening centers find children wearing headphones and turning the pages of a book to the tune of a bell. Emotion is strangely absent from their faces. With space at a premium, computers are often placed in foyers outside the classrooms, and I am always a bit disheartened to see young children disengaged from their peers socially and verbally, headphones firmly in place. Sometimes I feel a little old fashioned.

I see that reading and other specialized learning groups, although fully necessary if grade standards are to be met, can isolate the teacher and leave the rest of the children to work on their own. Teachers describe their inability to monitor and their concern that many children work without the benefit of their assistance. They may then be left to evaluate children's work by the quality of the finished product and cannot monitor the *process* of learning. The use of worksheets may become more common as a way to engage the larger group easily and independently, but they preclude the vital guided instruction that young children need as they gain new knowledge or practice new skills. I find this to be particularly true regarding the development of letter formation and writing mechanics, and believe that many bad habits become engrained as a result. My teacher colleagues also express frustration at the limits imposed upon the art of their profession.

The *far senses* of vision and hearing are more heavily recruited in the primary classroom; however, as is discussed in Chapter 5, the *near senses*, which arise from the movement of the body and its interaction with the environment, are powerful, effective, and instructive. I once watched while the students of a skilled and creative first-grade teacher marched, jumped, sang, and clapped in a physical display of verbs. The child with whom I was working, who generally had difficulty with selective attention, was fully engaged and actually got it. In this wonderful lesson, his body was asked to help.

Occasionally, I provide in-service training regarding sensory and motor development and the connection to learning. During our discussions I encourage teachers to ask the following series of questions: "How can I teach this concept to the whole child?" "How can I teach writing without writing?" "How long can we leave pencils in the box?" I often initially sense anxiety regarding the anticipated time commitment, the chaos of movement activity, and subsequent inability to reestablish order. However, order is only occasionally lost and is never irretrievable. Movement sees to that by organizing the whole learning circuit and readying the child for yet more learning. There is an art to it. Children provide cues, and a wild escalation can be prevented with a gradual deceleration of motion using calming rhythms. Some activities are more organizing than others, as we will also discuss in Chapter 5. Once teachers are comfortable with the principles, the ideas flow like rain!

FINAL THOUGHTS

This chapter has begun to lay a foundation for collaborations on student factors, environmental components, and task demands as they interconnect to influence occupational performance in the educational environment. As discussed, movement is integral, not supplemental, to learning, and it has an influence in every learning foundation from attention to transfer, motivation to literacy, math to memory, and language to social competence.

A wide developmental range, inherent wiggliness, and a need for movement are the guaranteed hallmarks of the young child in school, and they earn an abiding place on the list of K–3 student factors. The concept of DAP applies throughout this level, and occupational performance can improve given due attention to the characteristics of environment and task demand. Conversely, teachers and OTs are afforded the opportunity to evaluate and eliminate unintended constraints on DAP or on the performance of an individual child when they access the link between movement and learning to provide a natural balance of student, environment, and task. With a consensus regarding the importance of the movement–learning link, teachers and OTs can begin the creative process of inventing alternative instructional activities that reflect the embodied nature of learning. These are explored in Chapter 6 of this book, "The Knowledge-Sharing Team in Action." First, however, we should add to our vocabulary of interrelated factors and turn to an examination of fine motor performance and demand in school as we continue to share knowledge—OT to teacher—in the next chapter concerning little hands.

3

Little Hands in School

The work of little hands can escape consideration during the design of early math and literacy programs. Yet, developing automaticity in fine motor ability, particularly concerning the grasp and controlled manipulation of a pencil, plays significantly in the balance of student factors, environmental components, and task demands. As knowledge is shared regarding hand function and the emergence and progression of drawing, one hope is for the mounting of a renewed and suitable awe in the fine motor components of learning and due reflection on the nature and pace of their own unique learning trajectory during the primary years.

THE MOTOR-SENSORY HAND

Little hands are amazing. Each hand consists of 27 bones, including 8 in the wrist. Each is activated by more than 40 muscles that either reside fully in the hand itself (intrinsic) or lie in the forearm with long tendons that pass through the wrist and attach within the hand (extrinsic). Both extrinsic and intrinsic muscles function as an integrated system, but contribute differently to biomechanical balance in task performance. The extrinsic muscles of the forearm serve position, stability, and power, whereas the intrinsic muscles in the hand are particularly suited to enable the repetitive, reciprocal, or sequential finger movements of refined dexterity. There are eight (sometimes nine) muscles attached to the thumb alone, which aid its premier role in opposability and diverse exploratory movement. It is the only digit that can rotate or swivel, allowing it maximal freedom in grasp and manipulation (Wilson, 1998). As Wilson describes, another form of opposition is actually uniquely human—the ability to bring the pinkie and ring fingers across the palm toward the base of the thumb. This subtle motion would not seem to be functionally significant, but indeed it provides for the ability to hold a tool in line with, rather than solely perpendicular to, the forearm. Thus, humans can wield a hammer or swing a golf club or a tennis racket, but they could not play satisfactorily with a chimpanzee.

The movement of the arm and hand is elegant and can appear perfectly fluid. Considering the astronomical number of possibilities for the trajectory of the limb in space, the position of joints, the force of grasp, and the coactivity of muscles, it would seem an impossible task to develop any degree of poise and grace. It is particularly miraculous when we find that there is actually no continuous body movement. Rather, every movement consists of a series of discontinuous and pulsatile, smaller but synchronized motions that turn off and on according to an internal timing mechanism (Melillo & Leisman, 2004). This strategy—the synchronization of oscillating movements within the muscles—reduces the demand on the nervous system by allowing it to go rhythmically offline and, thus, increasing the efficiency of motor activity. Postural muscles, which stabilize for movement, and hand muscles, which act on the environment, are not connected spatially, but are activated and coordinated together in a moment in time to create the perception of a single and continuous motion. It is brilliant and beautiful.

In using the hand for exploration and function, the young child is already distinguishing between power and precision grips and between the cooperative work of both hands together or the use of one hand alone. Precision grips place an object between thumb and fingers to pinch or manipulate, as in holding a needle and thread. They may recruit one or all of the fingers in concert with the opposing thumb. The power grip seeks to immobilize an object in the hand and generally uses the palm for support, although a *hook* grasp involved in carrying a bucket may not. Throwing a ball, picking up a full can, and pounding with a hammer all involve the power grip. It is fashioned when static force or stability is required, and it limits the manipulative engagement of the thumb and activates virtually all of the muscles of the forearm (Wilson, 1998).

An important point is that grip pattern is not solely dictated by the shape of the object, but by the goal of the individual and the demands of the task. The same tool may be held and moved in different ways, as when twiddling a pencil or using it to write. Grasp will be matched to the demands of the activity and can quickly change from precision to power grip as children prioritize elements of the task, despite the presence of more precise movement possibilities in their manipulative repertoire. How often, for example, have we seen a child switch to a whole-hand grasp of the crayon in order to quickly cover a large space on the paper? Precision of both grasp and product will be sacrificed in an effort to meet the demand for rapid coverage—a prioritized goal of the child. He or she will find, however, that the change of strategy carries a cost in energy because fatigue may quickly set in when using the power grip. A reversion to the use of a power grip to draw or print may also be evident when the academic task is challenging, when hand preference is not well established, or when the child is in need of more time in fine motor rehearsal.

IN-HAND MANIPULATION

By the time little hands reach elementary school, they are capable of great diversity in a range of maneuvers beyond the simple ability to grasp. They can accomplish, but have not yet mastered, the basics of in-hand manipulation—the ability to adjust an object within the hand for exploration or use—*after* the object has been grasped. In-hand manipulation involves precision grip and is defined as having the following three components (Pehoski, 1995):

1. *Translation* involves the movement of a small object from finger tips into palm or from palm back into finger tips. Gathering lunch money coins, counting math manipulatives, maneuvering a bead from palm onto a string, dropping a handful of pennies singly into a bank, or placing bingo chips onto the board may all involve this operation. When translating a group of objects, there is a separation of the two sides of the hand in performing separate functions (this will appear again during crayon and pencil prehension). Using your preferred hand, for example, pick up three pennies from the table, one at a time. As soon as one coin is in your palm, your pinkie and ring fingers hold it securely, while thumb, index, and middle fingers retrieve and manipulate the second coin. By the age of 5 1/2, children happily experiment with these back and forth maneuvers, although the holder side of the hand may get some help via a variety of sneaky but effective little compensatory strategies. Watch the children closely. When the task demand requires careful management of the object, they may try one of three approaches to avoid dropping the treasure. Often, the first likely trick is simply to bring the other hand in to assist. More subtly, however, they may pick up the object and move it quickly to the chest to manipulate it against a solid and stable body surface. Or, watching even more closely, you may observe children turning their hands upward after each object retrieval, thus allowing gravity, rather than manipulation, to drop the item into their palms. These strategies are all perfectly smart and illustrate the ongoing experimentation and rehearsal that takes place, even after children appear to have mastered a particular manipulative skill.

2. *Rotation* of objects in the hand occurs with simple or complex sequential movement depending on the task. Simple rotation allows a jar lid to be opened. Complex rotation twirls a pencil in the hand or fully turns a small peg over before placing it into a hole. The most mature rotary movements are demonstrated by age 6 1/2 and are mastered gradually over time. The teacher who is alert to the rotary requirements of object manipulation can strategically place a crayon or pencil on the desk to facilitate prehension. For example, if the pencil point is facing away from the child, he or she will have to pick it up using complex

rotation to reposition it for use and may or may not be successful. If, alternatively, the pencil is placed on the table with its point directed toward the child's belly, a *simple* rotation will elevate the pencil into place. A minor change in environment and task demand thus influences the performance outcome.

3. In *shift* maneuvers, the thumb is highly active in creating linear movement, as in separating the pages of a book or performing *pencil push-ups* (walking the fingers up and down the shaft of the pencil). If it is not well established in the child's repertoire, he or she may be observed using both hands to position the pencil or maintaining an awkward finger position on the writing tool. When shift is present, the child will adjust the pencil in hand, moving fingers automatically toward the tip.

The full complement of in-hand manipulation skills is generally present by age 6 1/2. After that, no new skills emerge, but all become more efficient and automatic with practice over time, and the teacher will observe considerable variation in fine motor ability among children in the primary grades. The ability to be nimble with diverse prehensions, however, assumes that the goal activity presents the appropriate challenge, with the elements of student, environment, and task in balance. While the child is still experimenting with manipulative strategies, a simple output requirement (unstructured coloring or play with small materials) may be most appropriate. If a complex academic task is required (composing a sentence), watch for changes or adaptations in grip or in pressure on the tool. Small manipulatives are everywhere. I collect them at home and prowl through office supply, hardware, craft supply, and even plumbing stores to find likely treasures. The following are some ideas for the K–3 collection:

- Plastic coins and banks (boxes with slits in the top)
- Empty plastic spice jars with shaker tops (Include a supply of small wooden pegs or cut the sharp tips off of toothpicks to create an inexpensive peg board!)
- Rubber stamps, puzzles with knobs, mini puzzles, stickers
- Containers of all shapes and sizes
- Wrapping paper and ribbons
- Small plastic animals and vehicles
- Tweezers, including the small scissor-type
- Mini erasers and shaped buttons
- Small stencil kits with dabbing sponges
- Hole punches and clay shape cutters

- Threaded plastic pipes
- Mini wood craft construction kits
- Junk mail for pretending to fill out important forms

WHICH LITTLE HAND?

"Which hand does he use?" This would seem a fairly straightforward question, but there is disagreement about the definition of handedness, and its classification is actually a bit tricky. We are the most *lateralized* of beings, and a strong hand preference is considered to be uniquely human, just like language and extensive tool use (Wilson, 1998). We are "lopsided," so to speak.

Over the centuries, experts from a variety of fields have offered diverse speculation regarding the reason for the higher prevalence of right-hand dominance in the world's population (e.g., Carlyle, 1871, as cited in Annett, 1998). This includes the ancestral tendency for mothers to carry infants in their left arms (over their hearts) or for warriors to protect their hearts with their shields. In either case, the right hand is freed for use. Alternatively, early throwing behavior may have favored right-hand use, which emerged from the timing and sequencing precision of the *left* brain in monitoring this survival action on the right side (Annett, 1998; Wilson, 1998). Whatever the reason, the left hemisphere of the brain controls both speech and right-hand use in most people. It becomes trickier, however, biologically speaking because some people have a different pattern of asymmetry for language. It may be specialized in the right brain or both hemispheres, but either way these people tend toward right-hand dominance. Even most left handers have a left-brain specialization for speech.

Annett (1998) hypothesized that hand preference is stable with age and time, but that it is a continuous variable and is not accurately defined as left or right or either/or. Many people use a mix of left and right hands, depending on the action. Some research is based on hand preference for writing, in which case there is a reported 90% preference for right-handedness and 10% for left (Annett, 1998; Noroozian, Lotfi, Gassemzadeh, Emami, & Mehrabi, 2002). This is not a complete picture, however, because social prejudice historically biases toward right-handed writing. Although this influence has waned culturally, it was prevalent in the United States until the 1930s when childhood stuttering was feared to result from the social pressure of forced use of the right hand. Thus, there is a lower incidence of left-handed writers in our oldest population.

Other researchers determine laterality by measuring speed and precision in observed dexterity tasks, resulting in a measure of *relative hand skill*. Interestingly, approximately 16% of the population is faster with their left hand on these refined and timed tasks (Annett, 1998). Bear with me here.

Only two thirds of this subgroup is left handed for *writing* (bringing us back to approximately 10% of the total), possibly reflecting a lingering influence of social bias toward the right hand for this activity, but indicating a higher incidence of left-handedness than is determined by handwriting alone. Measures of hand preference on a variety of tasks are best observed directly, as self-report for handedness is notoriously unreliable and generally results in an either/or classification based primarily on preference for writing. When asked to perform a variety of other dexterous actions, many people are surprised to find that they have some mixed-hand use.

In Annett's research with children and adults, more stable proportions are derived from combined evidence of self-report, observed behavior, and relative hand skill in timed dexterity tasks, resulting in a three-fold classification. Those who are consistently left handed (no right-hand preference) are approximately 4% of the population. Consistent right handers (no left) make up 66% of the population. Mixed handers are 30% of the population and are further subclassified with weak to moderate preference along the continuum. For writing, the proportion of left handers is consistent at 10%.

How early is hand preference evident in the child? Interestingly, other indices of laterality can be observed quite early. The neonate's preference for head turning to the right is considered to be a strong predictor of later hand preference (Fagard, 1998). Spontaneous and targeted arm and hand movement and hand-to-mouth behavior is also seen more frequently on the right in infants. After the age of 7–8 months, right-hand preference is common for reaching and grasping. Although this tendency remains strong, variability and flexibility are common, and hand preference is not generally considered pronounced until the ages of 2–4 years.

We often think that *bimanual* manipulation is a precursor to handedness; however, complementary hand use (in which the hands play different active roles) is a later skill when compared with the emergence of hand preference in unilateral reach and grasp (Fagard, 1998). This makes sense when considering the greater synchrony and the simultaneous but different actions of each hand when using both together. Thus, the nondominant hand is actually considered to be specialized in its own way, primarily in stabilizing and in anticipating the spatial orientation of an object that will be acted on by the dominant hand (Wilson, 1998). Envision, for example, having to glue a broken teacup back together. Note how your nondominant hand turns the pieces actively for visual inspection and positions and holds them at just the right angle to await the precise work of the dominant hand. Imagine the calculations of time and space that are involved in managing the complementary movements of both hands in this single bimanual task.

Although most children will show a strong tendency for hand preference by the time they reach kindergarten, some continue to vacillate, and this is increasingly problematic for the child who is launched directly into literacy production activities at this early age. The refined control necessary for handwriting is dependent on specialization in one hand and support with the other, and the child who switches back and forth is at a distinct disadvantage. We know that learning is not effortful when the child is ready, but learning that writing is too hard may result in frustration and refusal behavior.

Switching between left and right hands for tool use does not necessarily indicate an absence of established hand preference. Rather, it can sometimes be evident in the child who has not yet developed mature *prehension* and who searches for a more comfortable grasp or who fatigues easily. An assessment of observed relative hand skill will often reveal the dominant hand, and simple modifications to materials or task will relieve this child. An OT may recommend some of the following strategies for a teacher to use:

- For the "switching" child *with* established hand preference but inefficient grasp:
  - Prioritize the process of tool use rather than the product.
  - Prioritize the development of prehension through the use of small manipulatives and the use of short crayon pieces on a vertical drawing surface.
  - Increase unencumbered fine motor rehearsal time through the availability of dramatic play materials, assembly toys and tools, or the opportunity to *disassemble* old gadgets.
  - Modify the task to reduce complexity and subsequent tension. For example, have this child circle or *stamp* a correct response (rather than copy a word) or paste a sequence of pictures (rather than produce a sentence). Literacy building need not await efficient grasp and may require a pencilless approach.
  - Reduce the work load to prevent fatigue and frustration, especially for the second and third graders whose writing demands are greater.
  - Use *worker hand* and *helper or holder hand* terminology (e.g., "Super! You picked up the crayon with your *worker* hand!" "I like how your *holder* hand is holding the paper down.")
- For the "switching" child without established hand preference:

- Encourage play on the floor; color or look at books while lying on tummy.

- Reduce the use of specialized tools (e.g., tear rather than cut; use letter stamps rather than pencil, use dictation or scribing).

- Modify academic tasks and workload.

- Place materials at the child's midline on the table so that he or she will make a choice. (Placing them on one side or the other may result in the use of "right hand on the right side" and "left hand on the left side.")

- Hang some toys on the wall (e.g., foam peg boards). The child's holder hand is required to stabilize the toy, and the worker hand may emerge. Provide materials that require complementary hand use (e.g., jars with twist-top lids, small penny banks, assembly toys).

- Ask the family about the child's hand preference during less demanding tasks such as toothbrush or spoon use. Have the child hammer with a toy hammer (a strong predictor of relative hand skill), and ask the OT for other ideas in determining the child's laterality. Be cautious about using ball skills as an indicator of hand preference. Right-handed children almost always throw with their right hand; left handers are less consistent with throwing and sometimes also use their right hand. Kicking is strongly associated with the throwing side (Wilson, 1998).

- Be sensitive to cultural preferences for right-hand use. Negotiate with the family. If parents express a desire for right-handedness (and they often share this information if the environment is safe and nonjudgmental), I am always careful to ask permission for the child to use his left hand with the pencil.

THE PENCIL IN HAND

Mechanically, the use of a pencil is about as lateralized as a task can be, and time allowed for the establishment of hand preference as a prerequisite is not a luxury. Pencil grasp and pencil *use* require the understanding of subtle differences having everything to do with the student–environment–task interplay. The *dynamic tripod*, considered to be a mature pencil grasp, is not a particularly complex prehension. It employs only a simple muscle synergy (among the first to emerge developmentally) in which all of the grasping fingers flex and extend simultaneously. Whereas the whole movement is sometimes called intrinsic because it involves the manipulation of an object within the hand, the grasp itself is managed by *both* intrinsic and extrinsic *musculature* (Manoel & Connolly, 1998). Over time, writers gain command of the combined components, including finger flexion and extension, which provide for minor reaching in the production of vertical pencil strokes, subtle movement of the wrist for forming loops, and relocation of the whole arm as it steers the pencil horizontally either for drawing or for letter and word spacing. The dynamic tripod is motorically efficient and economical and permits stability and precision while enabling the conservation of energy over time (see Figure 3.1).

In the dynamic tripod grasp, the two sides of the hand are fully separated with pinkie and ring fingers stabilizing against the paper and thumb, index, and middle fingers in active engagement on the tool itself. The pencil rests on the middle finger, but the pad of this digit is sometimes also on the pencil without consequence. The forearm is resting on the table, and the wrist is slightly cocked away from the surface. The pencil rests lightly against the back of the web, and fingers are relaxed in their movement.

Many children, particularly little girls, come to school fully prepared to use a pencil with precision and without the need for conscious monitoring. It is likely that they are already adept in their use of the dynamic tripod grasp, which tends to emerge between the ages of 4 and 6 1/2 years, and that their fine motor abilities are generally more advanced than their little boy peers. This age range for acquisition, however, anticipates the continuing variability of grasp patterns in the primary grades.

I mentioned pencil *use* as having different considerations than pencil prehension alone. I did so to call attention to the demands of task in the

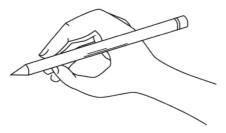

Figure 3.1. Dynamic tripod grasp with open web space.

evaluation of occupational performance within the early educational curriculum at the level of core instruction. The following are the subtleties:

- For children with typical motor abilities, the tripod pencil prehension is not a complex grasp.

- In-hand manipulation skills, which may not fully emerge until first grade and mature over a longer period of time, render the adjustment of the pencil in hand more challenging during task application. In research, for example, translation and rotation skills were found to be particularly significant predictors of handwriting scores (Cornhill & Case-Smith, 1996).

- Other factors play a role in the use of the pencil during functional application, including fine motor planning and visual-motor integration (these are discussed in Chapter 4). Importantly, writing specifically taxes the neurodevelopmental, linguistic, working memory, and executive skills of young children and bears heavily on the task of text production using a writing tool in the hand. In short, pencil grasp is a motor act and handwriting with a pencil is also a language task.

Returning to the topic of grasp, it is always wise to review the placement of little fingers on the pencil before beginning academic application. I generally look for the ability to make the "okay" sign with the fingers. Many teachers use the bird beak or alligator finger analogies. What the teacher will want to see is an *open web space* formed by the circle created by thumb and index finger. When the web space is open, refined movement is generated and the shoulder is relaxed. The term *static tripod grasp* simply means that the child places fingers in tripod formation on the pencil, but that movement is generated from the forearm and shoulder, whereas finger engagement is limited. It is slightly less mature, but typically it transitions easily to the dynamic version of the tripod grasp.

Children tend to experiment with and qualitatively modify their pencil grasp as late as age 12, and variations of the dynamic tripod are common (Ziviani, 1983). Younger children show greater variability within a task, which is a testament to the natural motor inconsistency that precedes a stable pattern during learning. Invariance of motor pattern, as automaticity increases, eventually becomes adaptive in freeing cognitive resources for higher level processing during the writing task (Greer & Lockman, 1998).

Pencil size and shape do not appear to influence drawing or writing for the typically developing child (Oehler et al., 2000), although teachers may wish to provide options for children, and OTs frequently experiment with a variety of writing tools for children with motor disabilities. Natural variations in grasp can be anticipated for much larger implements, such as markers, and are not a concern (Burton & Dancisak, 2000).

Transitional or modified grip configurations may not appreciably affect performance in the short term. Sometimes the thumb is placed against the side of the index finger (*lateral tripod*), wrapped over both the top of the pencil and index finger (or tucked under the index finger), and the forearm either resting or not resting on the table. Whatever this may be called, the decisive feature is a closure (partial or complete) of the open web space and a consequent limitation in the precision of intrinsic hand movement (see Figures 3.2 and 3.3).

The lateral tripod is a minor and common variation and is also considered to be an acceptable alternative configuration. The more closed the web space, however, the greater the concern for fatigue over time. Observing a closed grasp while out in my community, I have been known to ask store clerks (typically under the age of 30) whether their hand tends to fatigue during the day. Often I am greeted with a resounding "Yes!" Although writing legibility may not be noticeably affected, fatigue over time can be more likely, in my experience, although this is yet to be confirmed in formal studies. If detected early, a simple commercially available pencil grip will open the web space for more relaxed pencil use. Beyond the second grade, I find that children's grasps are much less amenable to change. It is notable at this point that the research is also variable on the relationship between pencil prehension and handwriting speed and legibility (see Chapter 4, "When Little Hands Write"). One observation of the characteristics of the research samples over time does seem to reflect an increasing prevalence of atypical grasps in school-age populations (Dennis & Swinth, 2001), a finding consistent with my own observations and of anecdotal reports by many of my teacher colleagues. Therefore, although this question continues to be explored, I would advocate for explicit instruction to students and ongoing monitoring regarding the placement of the pencil in hand.

It is also important to watch for the position of the thumb. It should be nicely rounded to achieve the "okay" sign and to allow for movement at all

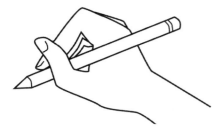

Figure 3.2. Lateral tripod grasp with partial closure of web space.

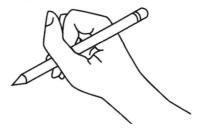

Figure 3.3. Thumb wrapped over pencil for full closure of web space.

the joints. If it is locked into a straight position (sometimes reflecting low muscle tone and consequent reduction of stability at the base of the thumb), one of two variations is likely to occur. First, the pencil may wave wildly upright in the air and tension will be felt in the forearm. Or, second, the index finger will curl high on the pencil with the other fingers spread evenly to its tip. In this grasp, the pinkie and ring fingers, which generally provide a supporting role, are both touching the pencil near its point (see Figure 3.4). I see this grasp most frequently in little boys. It is generally not transitional, but rather dysfunctional, and it is very difficult to change without specific intervention strategies. Although I am not familiar with any research in this area, I cannot help but note the similarity of this grasp to the grip used on some handheld computer gaming devices and may recommend a reasonable limitation of this activity, particularly in the youngest students.

A full *palmar*, or whole-hand grasp, with thumb pointing up or down is typical of a toddler and indicates a lack of motor readiness to use the tool for the most refined tasks. Flexible engagement of the fingers is notably absent in this grasp because they are tucked into the palm in a classic power grip. This child is best immersed in the process of tool use with a limited prioritization on product. The developmental age of a kindergartner can span within a 4-year range and not all children are ready to manage the motor requirements of academic work. The observation of this prehension requires the flexibility of the education team and a willingness to modify materials or task or both. The following are recommendations for correcting the whole-hand grasp (if a child in question receives occupational therapy, ask the child's OT for recommendations).

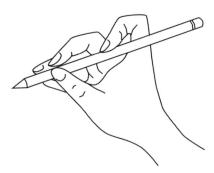

Figure 3.4. Thumb locked into straight position.

- Provide crayon pieces of about 1 1/2 inches in length. This may take some convincing, as children may not want to appear different from peers, but it is definitely worth a try at school and at home. A whole-hand grasp is not possible on such small pieces, and use of the fingers will be encouraged.

- Provide lots of opportunity to color on a slanted or vertical surface. Provide an easel or tape graffiti paper to the wall and encourage unstructured experimentation with the small crayons or chalk. The vertical orientation also encourages the forearm to rest on the surface, thus cocking the wrist and bringing fingers into a more natural tripod configuration.

- On the table, provide a mini easel by placing paper on a large three-ring binder that slants toward the child.

- If some refined pencil work is inevitable, allow the child to use a sharp, short crayon for early letter formation. It is not necessary for all children to use pencils and markers, and the drag created by crayon on paper provides for some additional control of the tool in hand.

- Seriously consider alternative means in beginning written letter formation for the child with the most compromised pencil grasp. For example, children can use a self-inking stamp to place their names on their projects. The OT is likely to be involved in these cases and will recommend an individualized approach to the introduction of writing.

As the child's prehension matures, begin to experiment with commercially available pencil grips. OTs typically carry a variety of styles, and teachers might also wish to have some on hand. One caution, however, is that pencil grips need only be provided to those children who are struggling with the development of prehension. During trial periods, the teacher will still need to observe the child carefully, as it is not unusual to see a more mature grasp emerge on the grip, only to disappear again when task demand increases or the child fatigues over time. Children are very creative in wrapping little fingers tightly around pencil and grip alike. Finally, pencil grips are a *temporary* aid to prehension, unless otherwise prescribed by the OT. Remove the grip occasionally to determine the child's ability to manage the pencil without this assist. He or she should be able to maintain the more mature grasp for several minutes without reverting to a previous style. If not, pop the pencil grip back on and check again in a month or two.

Teachers will observe other variations in pencil prehension and may wonder whether further instruction or modifications are necessary. Again, acknowledging the natural tendency for young children to experiment, explicit instruction regarding grasp pattern is highly encouraged. The following review of five important principles of effective use of the tool for eventual writing will help with this decision:

1. Separation: Over time, the two sides of the preferred hand separate in function. Pinkie and ring fingers stabilize and support, but are generally not engaged in the manipulation of the pencil. Thumb, index, and middle fingers generate refined movement.

2. Web space: The "okay" sign, formed with thumb and index fingers, opens the web space and allows for freedom of finger movement. A closed web space limits or eliminates this freedom and forces a reliance on the power muscles of the forearm, which fatigue under the strain of small, repetitive motion.

3. Thumb: The thumb is curved, not straight and locked. A locked thumb further constrains refined motion and forces movement at other hand joints, which do not have the anatomical luxury of rotation and swivel in opposition during the production of small strokes of the pencil.

4. Teach and Review: Children pass through transitional phases of pencil prehension, and minor variations are normal and acceptable. It will be necessary, however, to review the elements of mature pencil grasp regularly in class, even through the third grade.

5. Task demand: A *one task fits all* approach may not address the right motor challenge for all children. Consider flexible approaches to instructional methods and materials.

THE USE OF SCISSORS

Cutting activities are fairly complex and require the specialization of one hand for management of the tool and use of the other for dynamic manipulation of the paper. When using scissors efficiently, the child's hand demonstrates smooth *grading* of the open and close cycles, and fingers and thumb move rhythmically and smoothly in a rounded position. If graded movement is lacking, the child's fingers will often be fully extended, and the scissors will slip to the base of the thumb. There are many ways to modify the motor demands of cutting for children who continue to struggle with this complex bilateral activity. The following strategies may help:

- For the most challenged child, increase the priority on process. Provide heavy bond paper (which allows greater control) and encourage the child to tear with fingers or cut random shapes. Help the child tape the shapes together into a favored form (e.g., car, plane, paper doll) to satisfy both child and parent in the desire for a product.

- Provide the child with partially completed projects or draw a bubble (bold marker line) around the primary outline to reduce the complexity of the cutting task and prevent the tears that fall when important parts are inadvertently cut off. Use a few spots of glue to attach thin paper copies onto heavy bond paper.

- If the child has difficulty picking up the scissors correctly, put your hand firmly over the blades and hold them down on the table. Make sure the larger hole is positioned correctly for thumb access. As the child reaches for the scissors, hold them down firmly until his or her fingers and thumb have found their way into both holes (see Figure 3.5). Then release the tool and allow the child to pick it up. This will limit the manipulative requirements for prehension of the tool, but still allow the child some needed trial-and-error practice. Placing the scissors into the child's hands eliminates this valuable rehearsal.

- If hand preference is not yet fully established, place scissors on the table at the child's midline and let him or her choose. As hand preference becomes more consistent, use *worker, helper,* or *holder* terminology (e.g., "I see you put the scissors in your *worker* hand!" "I like the way your *helper* hand is turning the paper!")

- Begin to provide additional sensation and heavy work to the emerging preferred hand. Allow these children to cut through corrugated paper or two layers of construction paper. Give them projects that require handheld hole punching or have them use children's pinking shears or craft scissors.

- If graded movement is not yet evident, provide *self-opening* scissors, which spring open and thus eliminate the need for the controlled cycling of open-and-close hand movement (see Figure 3.6). Self-opening scissors are available through academic supply stores or school and therapy specialty catalogs. They can also be made, if needed, by coiling a jumbo paperclip to create a spring and taping it to a regular pair of scissors. Keep several pairs on hand.

THE SENSORY-MOTOR HAND

The hand serves the child in performing goal-directed actions. However, it is also a precise sensory organ that both receives and seeks sensation and could not function in the world without the capacity to feel. Each hand has 17,000 sensory receptors that detect touch pressure, temperature, weight, vibration, joint position, texture, and shape (Forssberg, 1998) and that mediate a relationship between the nervous system and the external world (Mountcastle, 2005). The eye is better than the hand in determining spatial detail, but the hand is better than the eye in resolving small lapses of time (as in sensitivity to the frequency of vibration). Overall, regarding the ability to feed sensory information to the brain, the visual and auditory systems are considered to be relatively simple compared to the extensive sensory involvement of the hand!

Manipulation and manual exploration of objects is a significant source of information for children whose tactile abilities are maturing rapidly. The

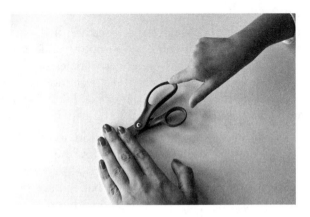

Figure 3.5.   Facilitating a child's grasp with scissors.

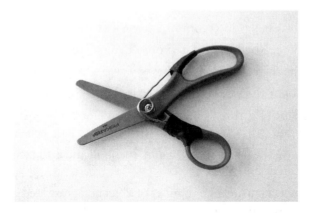

Figure 3.6. Homemade self-opening scissors.

ability to interpret the attributes and identity of common objects through manipulation without the aid of vision is called *haptic perception*. It forms one foundation for the hand's role in the construction of knowledge and is quite within the ability range of the 5-year-old child (Stilwell & Cermak, 1995). In relation to the movement–learning link, movement or manipulation with the hands is the key to haptic perception. Without movement, the sensory receptors in the hand begin to shut off and no longer contribute to the construction of knowledge. Without movement, the hand becomes insensitive. Hold, for example, a penny in your palm and do not explore it. It will not take long before you barely notice that it is there, just like the ring on your finger. The moment your hand flickers, awareness will return. Recognition of objects through haptic perception seems uncomplicated, but the exact mechanism by which the spatial and temporal input from the moving hand is instantaneously integrated to provide an awareness of "the whole" continues to be an unresolved problem for neuroscientists (Mountcastle, 2005). Amazingly, we can become immediately conscious of the identity of an object, but remain largely unaware of the astronomical amount of information involved in the *process* of feeling it.

Because haptic perception is astonishingly rich in information, haptic recognition games represent an untapped but lucrative field of creative instructional strategies that can supplement traditional teaching activities in early math or literacy without the *need for pencil and paper*. They are equally instructive, but modify the components of task demand in the student–environment–task interplay. I use them frequently, even for older children who continue to produce letter and number reversals or are correcting letter formation errors. The following are some haptic recognition games for the child to play to support general core instruction.

- Sort shapes into containers without looking.
- Match the manipulated objects to the correct picture.
- Match textures or weights.
- Count the sides of a geometric shape and name it.
- Identify a three-dimensional letter or number held in hand.
- Turn the letter (e.g., *b/d/p*) in hand until it faces the correct direction.
- Give a partner the number of objects represented by the three-dimensional number held in hand.
- Name a word whose beginning or ending letter is the same as the one held in hand.
- Describe the function of the common object in hand.
- Take turns with peers to develop a "continuous story" based on the various objects in hand.
- Describe the attributes of the object in hand (e.g., short, cold, metal, curved) and wait until the peer with the matching object raises his or her hand (e.g., both are holding a paper clip).

Haptic perception is a natural supplement to conceptual and language development and is a powerful partner in visual-spatial information analysis. Vigorous debate continues regarding the issue of whether the visual processing system itself can be influenced, changed, or trained through cognitive or behavioral methods. Teachers and therapists, however, play a considerable role in *supporting* this domain through many effective educational strategies.

Visual-spatial information analysis, similar to haptic perception, allows the child to gather information from the environment and organize and integrate it with past experience for the construction of new learning. It requires more than vision and ocular-motor control and includes many capacities and abilities that are amenable to instruction. Children can indeed be taught to allocate their attentional resources, to visually and systematically scan spatial elements for relevant detail, and to sustain attention to task. Teachers are adept at designing visual memory and sequencing aids, including highlighting salient information in print, verbal retelling, and pattern recognition. They train young children in print awareness, including the spatial ordering of left–right and top–bottom orientation. They challenge the discrimination of subtle visual differences with pictures and symbols and facilitate compare and contrast ability through matching and categorization. They teach children daily about the organization and management of the spatial environment.

The *interpretation* of information, including visual-spatial, is a central feature of constructivist teaching methodology. Children construct their knowledge within the scaffolded learning activities of the classroom where meaning is derived from experience and action on the world, not only from the analysis of two-dimensional pictures and symbols, but also from the exploration of objects and three-dimensional space as well as with engagement in the organization and sequence of events and movement experiences in the daily life of the child at school. The teacher's role in the design of effective activities and a supportive environment is unmistakable. Haptic attention to shape, form, and detail through a recruitment of the sensory-motor hand undoubtedly adds yet another strategy to the teacher's toolbox in support of core instruction.

WHEN LITTLE HANDS DRAW

Children's drawings have been examined, studied, and researched for decades. They have represented a *printout* of the inner mental life of the child and a mirror of his or her emotional well-being (Golomb, 2004). Some early theorists subscribed to the maturational or, more specifically, a copyist viewpoint, which holds that the simplistic drawings of the young child (younger than 8 or 9 years) reflect an immature ability to conceptualize the world and deal logically with its spatial elements. This view assumes that the child strives to *copy* the world around him but is unsuccessful due to his immature cognitive, motor, perceptual, executive, or memory resources. In the maturational view, the adult's appreciation of realism is held as a standard by which the child's drawings are judged, and simple renditions are considered incomplete, inaccurate, or defective. Drawing stages, whether measured by product (the developmental acquisition of shapes); concept (fixed progression from scribbling to design); or process (progression through graphic production principles, such as top–bottom or left–right formation) are held as stable and rigid and are insensitive to external constraints. Thus, under these assumptions, the child's early graphic forms should not be modifiable, and the same "errors" should be evident across changes in instruction and task demand. Meaning is absent from the child's early graphic ventures in the maturational viewpoint.

Since the 1960s, researchers have awakened to the symbolic substance of the young child's drawings and have studied them as productions of a unique graphic domain of learning (Arnheim, 1974; Lewis, Russell, & Berridge, 1993; Thomassen, Meulenbroek, & Hoofs, 1992; Vinter, 1999). Over time, the maturational perspective has found less support in more recent findings of the dynamic influences of both internal and external attributes. Golomb (2004) outlined the major assumptions of this new perspective, which places greater emphasis on the meaning and significance of children's drawings. Children do not attempt to *copy* nature or to create a one–one correspondence with the object; rather, they try to *represent* it with an *acceptable equivalent* (Golomb, 2004, p. 29) That their markings can stand for something is an early discovery of the child. Young children, however, lack a graphic vocabulary and thus adhere to the principle of economy in the conveyance of meaning with the most basic of forms. Thus, as Golomb (2004) contends, their drawings are not "missing" anything; they are complete and economical renditions of the world that reveal vivid, although nascent, symbolic understanding.

The problem-solving nature of a curious and communicative mind grapples with a translation of the three-dimensional world into a two-dimensional plane. Rules of graphic production in a universal graphic language are present in developmental tendencies; however, variability, rather than rigidity, is the hallmark of progression. Symbolic meaning is evident even in the preschooler's strategic placement of scribbles with appropriate "body parts" (as verbalized by the child) aligning on a vertical axis from top to bottom. In addition, complex storylines can be revealed in children's running commentaries as they narrate their scribbles in fantasy. My own son, Cale, was a master of drawing commentary, and I specifically recall conferring with his teacher about it many years ago. Even as late as kindergarten, a mass of swirls and broad, rapid strokes, although absent of visible representation, were nonetheless the traces of exploding stars and rocket excursions to unknown and distant planets, as he happily described them.

Golomb (2004) described evidence both *for* developmental trend and *against* a fixed progression. Four particular lines of study have suggested that protracted maturation through scribbling phases is not always the case. First, children in remote South American and Arabian villages transition rapidly from experimental scribbling to representational human depictions, despite a lack of previous graphic experience. Second, children with congenital blindness (probably informed by tactile sensory exploration) can and do produce two-dimensional human equivalents when provided with drawing materials, even without prior scribbling. Thus, presymbolic markings, although valuable, are not fixed precursors. Third, Golomb's own experiments reveal the dynamic interplay of child factors, environmental components, and task demand in the emergence of representational drawing that is independent of previous experience and practice. For example, when verbally encouraged to add parts, the young child will do so with correct spatial relationship, suggesting that scaffolding can mobilize the child's capabilities beyond his independent efforts. The fourth line of study notes that young scribblers will often add recognizable body parts, such as trunk and legs, to a head or face drawing offered by the examiner. Belying a "faulty" perception, the adult's encouragement for detail will overcome the child's adherence to economy.

This sensitivity to external cues and task demand is also seen as a result of the specificity of instructions provided for drawing. The young child's tendency to produce the *canonical* view of a familiar object (e.g., a mug with the handle to the side), regardless of the child's actual view of the object, once corroborated the maturational perspective that children are bound by intellectual, rather than visual, realism and tend to draw their *understanding* of the world and not what they *see* in the world. Lewis and colleagues (1993) found, however, that when 5-year-old children are given increasingly more specific direction ("draw exactly what you see from where you are sitting"), their depictions of mug and handle position become accordingly more realistic and, therefore, less canonical. This finding further questions the maturational viewpoint and is informative to teachers and OTs who collaborate on educational strategies in support of core instruction and whose verbal guidance to children may entice a more elaborate performance outcome. Drawing, therefore, is open to scaffolding.

A general rule of the drawing progression is the advancement from simple to more complex formations, which operates not only by the refinement of dexterity and visual-motor-spatial ability, but also by children's own increasing need to clarify the meaning of their work. Rooted in the representational origins of drawing, children begin to differentiate their ambiguous early efforts with new strategies as they are discovered and added to the graphic vocabulary.

By the time children reach kindergarten, assuming their typical development and opportunity with drawing materials, they are likely to have auditioned every conceivable form of scribble from horizontal and vertical lines to squiggles, zigzags, and spirals. By age 3, they have discovered the single closed circle, which evokes interpretation and launches them into the world of representational shape. By closing the figure and creating an interior space, children have at their artistic disposal the foundation of design with its inherent potential to transform into any number of objects in the world—real or imagined.

Already at this point, children are becoming obedient to graphic production rules for lines and circles, although variability is an ally and allows the adaptive freedom to solve problems of task demand and the conveyance of meaning. Over time, experimental variability will decrease, which is an equally adaptive solution favoring automaticity and the prioritization of higher cognitive and executive processing.

THE NUTS AND BOLTS OF LINES AND SHAPES

Although variable, there is a progression to children's drawing and prewriting graphic production. It is flexible and does not represent a fixed sequence or rigid timetable. Based on the research of Beery and Beery (2004) and others (Braswell & Rosengren, 2000; Scheirs, 1990; Vinter, 1999), as well as my personal observations, this section offers a general guideline of these graphic forms.

Vertical and horizontal lines are generally *imitated* at ages 2 and 2 1/2, respectively, and copied at ages 2 years 10 months and 3 years, respectively (Beery & Beery, 2004). Children imitate forms that are demonstrated to them. They copy forms that are presented as a two-dimensional model but are not demonstrated by peer or adult. The ability to imitate generally precedes the ability to copy.

Biomechanical constraints of the arm and hand tend to favor the increasing consistency in top–bottom production for the vertical stroke (Braswell & Rosengren, 2000), although, in my experience, bottom–up formation is not uncommon in the early grades. Often, the bottom–top stage, which may be evident in 2- to 3-year-olds, is protracted for children who have a limited command of the adaptive response, narrow strategy repertoires and do not easily transition away from familiar patterns. Children with autism, for example, may persist in this and other initial action strategies and may require instruction for directional stroke production in preparation for letter formation. Hand preference does not seem to have a strong influence on the direction of the vertical line at any age.

Young children (ages 4 and 5 years) prefer to attach their lines to an *anchor* (a previously drawn form) and will produce the rays of a sun from the circle outward. Anchoring declines with age and eventually gives way to the top–bottom vertical form. Older children and adults, therefore, will draw the top sun rays toward the circle and the bottom rays away from the circle (Braswell & Rosengren, 2000). The strategy of anchoring is in conflict with top–down letter formation toward a baseline and may present an obstacle for the kindergartner who is printing on a baseline.

The *horizontal line* is the only stroke that differentiates between left- and right-hand preference (Scheirs, 1990). Although there may be some variability in the youngest children (age 2 years), the right-handed child will tend to produce this stroke from left to right and the left-handed child from right to left. Instructional and cultural influences, however, are also at work. Arabic children, for example, will produce script, including individual letter strokes, from right to left. Interestingly, Hebrew children, who also begin script on the right of the page tend to produce individual letter strokes from left to right (Braswell & Rosengren, 2000).

Closed circles are often copied at age 3, shortly after they are imitated (Beery & Beery, 2004). Regardless of hand preference, 3- to 5-year-olds may produce them with a clockwise stroke beginning at the bottom. After the age of 5 years, the counterclockwise circle increases in frequency; however, variability is certainly evident for a few more years. For example, Braswell and Rosengren found that the counterclockwise circle was established in only 62.5% of 7-year-old children. First- and second-grade teachers, therefore, may continue to encounter the initial procedure in some children, and monitoring for letter formation will be necessary. Shape and letter formation can be rehearsed in many ways, and circles can be practiced while producing pumpkins on a fence or apples on a tree.

At approximately 4 years of age, children will begin to combine horizontal and vertical strokes to copy a *cross*; they will copy a *square* later at approximately 4 1/2 years (Beery & Beery, 2004). Production of the square beginning at the top left corner and proceeding downward and around with a continuous stroke is fairly consistent from age 4 or 5 years and represents a developmental tendency called *threading*. This continuous line strategy in which the pencil is never raised from paper peaks and is dominant at approximately 6–7 years and is commonly used for closed shapes and contours (Vinter, 1999). At this age, many children will also experiment with the same action pattern to produce a human figure having a single, continuous outline. Whereas the threaded production of the square persists to adulthood, threading used as an experimental strategy for other contours declines in strength after age 8 when meaning is best conveyed by the segmentation of parts. The continuous line square tends to override other line production strategies, including the top–bottom vertical and left–right horizontal.

Triangles, which become graphically available after the emergence and combination of oblique lines, are copied by about 50% of children at age 5 years 3 months (Beery & Beery, 2004). There is, however, considerable variability in formation procedure continuing throughout the K–3 years. A child's comfort with the production of oblique lines plays a role in early representational drawing and letter formation, and avoidance of the diagonal will not only influence the appearance of roofs on houses, but also of capital letters, such as A, K, M, and N, as well as the ability to conform to the requirements of slanted alphabets (e.g., D'Nealian style).

WHEN SHAPES COME TO LIFE

The production of a closed circle at age 3 is closely followed by the endowment of animate details. A *global human* (one lacking trunk and limbs) soon transforms into the classic *tadpole* (an ambiguous frontal depiction in which arms and legs sprout from a central circle, bounding both head and body in a single stroke) (see Figure 3.7). The tadpole is graphically logical and economical to perfection, an ingenious rendition that earns the 3- to 4-year-old child immediate praise and encouragement from adults. Any further elaboration is offered verbally, not graphically, by the child, and the inherent ambiguity of this simple figure eventually drives the artist to differentiate with additional detail. Thus, graphic production begins to serve meaning through defining features, such as hair length or simple clothing style. Early efforts to enhance complexity, however, will be met with the old dilemma of translation to the two-dimensional plane. *Transparency,* or the tendency to overlap outlines so that one figure is seen through the other, is common for the kindergartner and represents a workable solution to the dimension problem until other strategies are discovered. As graphic vocabulary increases throughout the K–3 level, children will learn to use detail, shading, color, segmentation of parts, spatial orientation, and the occlusion of hidden parts to further support intent and meaning. As oblique lines enter the graphic repertoire, concepts such as movement and action can be portrayed with slants in trunk and limb direction (Golomb, 2004).

THE ROLE OF PRIVATE SPEECH

Our ability to collaborate on the most effective strategies for children requires a mutual understanding of the contributions of all learning domains within a specific educational activity. The role of *private speech* in children's

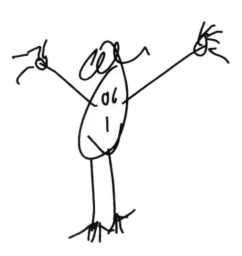

Figure 3.7. Tadpole figure.

drawing provides such an opportunity to examine the relationship between the drawing task and the child's self-regulatory or metacognitive efforts and should not be overlooked as a window into the child's management of task demand. Private speech is talk that is spontaneous and self-directed, serves a self-regulatory and attentional function in young children, and reveals cognitive problem solving as it is immediate and ongoing. It is quite common and is comprised of 20%–60% of the classroom language of children between the ages of 3 and 10 years (Berk, 2001). Berk also notes that private speech is more abundant, although less effective, for self-regulation in children with attention-deficit/hyperactivity disorder (ADHD).

Two founding principles become evident in the observation of children's private speech. First, cognitive resources for new learning are available to the extent that they are dispersed primarily to higher level processes as fluency or automaticity is established in the lower level processes. Second, student factors, environmental components, and task demands are tightly interrelated. Investigating the responses of first, third, and fifth graders, Matuga (2004) studied the variants of private speech and their relationship to changes in task demand in realistic versus make-believe drawing activities.

Two forms of audible private speech were revealed (along with inaudible muttering) and were used either to accompany the task (singing, labeling, or running commentary) or to employ metacognitive strategies for planning, monitoring, and self-evaluating. The combined metacognitive verbalizations were composed of 47% of total private speech. Overall, the findings suggest that children talk to themselves more frequently when the task is more creative and less formulaic. As drawings of familiar objects, such as person or house, are rehearsed and automatized, they impose little challenge to the working child. However, when familiar action strategies are restructured for novelty and creative idea generation, self-regulatory and attentional requirements are heightened. Task demand is again highly influential, constraining student factors in the cognitive domain. Importantly, children with average or low creative ability were more reliant on self-regulatory private speech than highly creative children.

STEP-BY-STEP DRAWING AND OTHER STRATEGIES

Although step-by-step drawing is fairly constrained regarding creativity, it can be a valuable instructional exercise to facilitate visual-motor ability and initial drawing strategies for children who struggle to generate ideas and action plans. Children love to arrive at a product that enhances their independence, not to mention their motivation and personal satisfaction. I have had great success with some very reluctant writers and artists in "publishing" original comic books based on step-by-step models. Creativity and confidence simply emerge from a different direction in this scaffolded drawing approach.

I also use step-by-step drawing for the development of both visual and auditory memory. Having presented the child (or group) with a simple shape sequence (e.g., circle-square-triangle), I remove the stimulus and the children draw from memory. As they become more proficient, we progress to simple representational drawings and then to letters or words, depending on age and ability. Auditory memory is enhanced when a simple series of shapes or letters is dictated, and children produce them independently. In addition to sequences, I incorporate spatial concepts in my instructions. For example, "Put a circle on the top of the page and a square on the bottom," or "Make a circle and put an x in the center." These strategies support learning and problem solving and are used for purposes other than creative drawing.

The visual-spatial components of drawing can also be supported with the use of alternative materials, such as playdough or construction paper parts. I often have children construct human figures and simple representational shapes (e.g., house or car) from paper or magnetic pieces. Thus, the graphic production rules, such as top–bottom sequencing and simple–complex progression are explored without pencil in hand.

Drawing-on-dictation, as described by Golomb (2004), is effective in expanding the child's application of detail. This method involves simply suggesting additional parts or having the child dictate them to you to support learning. The language exchange can be augmented by inspiring the thinking process with the use of more abstract leading questions. For example, if ears are missing on the figure, try asking "How will he hear me?" If hands are missing, say "How can he hold his spoon?"

FINAL THOUGHTS

Our collaborative toolbox is filling up, and we are arming the education team with new information as we plan strategies and evaluate the balance of student, environment, and task. We have reviewed student factors, including the development of in-hand manipulation, the complexity of hand preference, variations in grasp, and the developmental tendencies of graphic production. In support of successful educational performance, we have explored environmental components, including materials to facilitate dexterity, the features of writing tools and scissors, and other materials that encourage effective tool use. We have addressed the modification of task demand in the presence of ambiguous hand preference or immature prehension and have introduced haptic perception and drawing strategies to support concept and language development, memory and attention, and idea generation. Our treatment of drawing is not complete, however. In Chapter 4, we further examine the drawing–writing link and its implications for K–3 education.

4

When Little
Hands Write

If any province of learning begs the integration of shared knowledge among all members of the education team, it is handwriting. Difficulty with this single educational task is one of the primary reasons for referral to the school-based occupational therapist (OT), and underlying dysfunction in fine motor ability is often the assumed culprit. Yet, the assessment and remediation of handwriting challenges in young children is necessarily a collaborative effort to discover all sources of barrier to the writing process, and the most cogent analysis draws from a range of constituent learning domains. The ultimate goal is not legible handwriting, but the successful communication of ideas with compositional fluency and quality. At the level of core instruction, collaboration on the issue of handwriting places primary focus on a strong writing foundation and the prevention of many writing obstacles.

In my informal conversations with teachers, I often say something that surprises them, which is "You know as much as I know about handwriting." Putting words on the page is not solely, and often not primarily, a visual-motor activity. It is, first and foremost, a linguistic exercise to which neuro-developmental, linguistic, and cognitive elements contribute concurrently (Abbott & Berninger, 1993; Wakely, Hooper, de Kruif, & Swartz, 2006). The discovery of correlations between reading and writing have, since the 1980s, inspired the recommendation by many researchers to teach these two literacy skills together. Thus, the introduction of more formalized writing expectations has filtered downward in the K–3 curriculum to the developmental level at which fine and visual-motor skills are their most variable. To follow the rationale for this contemporary practice and to examine the link between teacher and OT knowledge in the area of handwriting, reading and writing research is addressed first here.

THE READING–WRITING CONNECTION

At one time, writing was primarily seen through developmental lenses. Children scribble first, imitate simple lines next, and eventually print letters. Spelling develops from phonetic representations to the integration of orthographic rules. Reading and writing were formerly viewed as separable learning tasks, with reading viewed as the foundation and predecessor of writing behavior. In the design of instructional and intervention strategies, the developmental approach made it practical for teachers and OTs to go their separate ways in understanding and explaining children's writing.

These two literacy components, however, have most recently been found to be closely connected through a mutual dependence on shared cognitive processes and constrained by similar knowledge representations (Fitzgerald & Shanahan, 2000). If the overlap were complete, instructional separation would continue to make sense because generalization or transfer from reading to writing would occur easily. However, they are not. Reading and writing find a reciprocal relationship but are not perfectly aligned in learning. In Fitzgerald and Shanahan's (2000) example of spelling versus word recognition, the reader starts with the analysis of a *grapheme* (a letter or letter combination) and converts it to a single sound from a limited array of corresponding sounds. The writer, however, begins with the *phoneme* (smallest unit of sound) and engages in the task of choosing from an often nonintuitive variety of spellings.

Berninger and colleagues (Berninger, Abbott, Abbott, Graham, & Richards, 2002; Berninger et al., 2006) describe language behavior as alternatively received or expressed through four functional systems. The term *functional*, which in this case implies a connection, reflects the need for the brain to team up with sensory and motor systems for the communication of language. This is necessary because the brain itself has no output organ or method of its own. Instead, it receives language through the auditory and visual sensory systems for listening and reading and expresses language through the oral-motor and graphomotor systems for speaking and writing. Each of these functional systems—*language by ear, language by eye, language by mouth, and language by hand*—is organized uniquely and develops along a unique developmental trajectory. In addition, knowledge is often shared among them. The internal process is always linguistic, no matter which functional system is employed. Thus, it is no longer meaningful to isolate the functional language systems in evaluating and analyzing the skills and challenges of children's writing or to create artificial division between the knowledge and instructional intervention strategies of teachers and OTs in remediation for this highly integrated task.

Whether reading or writing is the more difficult skill is debated in the literature. Fitzgerald and Shanahan (2000), for example, posit that reading is somewhat easier, pointing to the phoneme–grapheme challenge for writers. Elbow (2004), however, considers writing the easier task because drawing precursors and invented compositional strategies allow the young child to pour all his thoughts and ideas onto the page, whereas the reader can only command what he has been specifically taught. Whatever the relative learning effort required for acquisition, consensus finds that considerable shared knowledge reasonably makes the combined instruction of these two literacy skill areas more efficient and effective for the young learner.

SHARED LINGUISTIC PROCESSES OF READING AND WRITING

Both readers and writers rely on a variety of receptive and expressive language processes, including phonological awareness, rapid automatic naming (RAN), orthographic knowledge, and semantics and syntax. *Phonological awareness* refers broadly to the manipulation of oral language sounds, including the ability to recognize and produce rhyme, blend or delete sounds, and segment words into syllables and syllable parts. *Phonemic awareness* is a component skill and more specifically involves the ability to recognize and manipulate or segment the *individual* sounds of words and to perceive and identify them as the same across words (Abbott & Berninger, 1993). The English language contains 26 letters, some of which are combined to create approximately 44 sounds or phonemes. For example, the word *bat* has three letters and three phonemes, /b/, /a/, and /t/. The word *boat* also has three phonemes when pronounced /b/, /o/, /t/, but it has an additional grapheme when written.

Young infants can discriminate language sounds, and children as young as 4 years can typically segment words into syllables. They do not, however, become consciously aware of phonemic segmentation as a consequence of engagement in spoken language and, therefore, must learn it explicitly (Vernon & Ferreiro, 1999). More precisely, as demonstrated in Vernon and Ferreiro's research, the acquisition of an alphabetic writing system appears to facilitate phonemic awareness, and the use of language-in-print can be a more effective instructional strategy than oral lessons alone. Furthermore, when children experiment with writing, they spontaneously engage in the analysis of speech, which strengthens their understanding of the structure of language sound and the connection between reading and writing.

Children with strong phonological skills can play with word sounds to verbally separate the two syllables of *cowboy*, to isolate the first sound of *map*, or to accurately substitute the sound /t/ for the sound /p/ to create a new word—*mat*. The ability to recognize and manipulate phonemes is considered to be a strong predictor of reading achievement in first grade and is often found to be a significant challenge for children with reading disabilities (Wolfe & Nevills, 2004).

Rapid automatic naming (RAN), or the ability to fluently name visually presented letters (with speed and accuracy), is also a reading precursor and is considered to be more important to reading success than the simple ability to recite the alphabet (Wolfe & Nevills, 2004). It is hypothesized that RAN reflects the efficiency of visual and phonological integration, and, along with phonemic awareness and orthographic coding, is one of the three most accurate predictors of later reading and spelling difficulties (Berninger et al., 2006).

Orthographic knowledge, which is functionally related to phonology, indicates the "knowledge and use of the specific letter patterns found in words" (Bowers & Ishaik, 2003, p. 148). It also reflects the ability to translate phonemes into graphemes. Thus, phonology involves pronunciation, whereas orthography refers to an understanding of spelling rules and patterns, as well as an awareness of the legal positions, frequencies, and combinations of graphemes in the written word (Apel, Wolter, & Masterson, 2006). For example, double consonants are common in the middle of a word (*better*), but they are not legal as an initial combination (*ffrog*).

Semantics refers to word, phrase, sentence, and text *meaning. Syntax* refers to word, phrase, and sentence *order* within the rules of grammar. Both are linguistic processes that have greater influence on writing in the intermediate grades (Wakely et al., 2006).

Although the terminology of linguistic processes is quite familiar to teachers, it may be introductory to OTs. In the next discussions of handwriting, an understanding of the place of linguistics in the writing process is necessary.

HANDWRITING IN THE WRITING PROCESS

Early in the acquisition of writing, developmental skills such as orthographic awareness and coding, fine motor ability, and visual-motor integration play heavily in learning and vary greatly from child to child. (The motor components of handwriting will be discussed later in the chapter.) In this section, their overall importance is noted in their foundational contribution to writing, including the confidence that is derived from the ability to put ideas to paper with joy and ease. The child who struggles significantly with the formative developmental components of writing, whether motor, linguistic, or cognitive, may disengage from the writing task or may refuse to formulate his or her ideas altogether.

Since 1980, writing has been described in terms of three higher level cognitive processes, planning, translating, and reviewing (Hayes & Flower, 1980), and pedagogical methods have incorporated the process writing approach. Process writing intends to release the author's voice by favoring an instructional focus on the higher level processes, rather than on discrete technical or mechanical skills such as grammar, spelling, and handwriting (Unger & Fleishman, 2004).

Hayes and Flower (1980) describe writing as a cognitive problem-solving task and, therefore, report several relevant neurocognitive functions that contribute to it. These include executive controls, attention, working memory, and language. The planning component of writing consists of idea generation and organization, along with goal setting. Translation involves the production of language that corresponds to ideas generated and stored in working memory; however, the specific components of the translation process were not defined. Reviewing includes reading and editing.

Abbott and Berninger (1993) have, as a result of further study, modified the original model for first through sixth grades to define the components of the translation process, which is missing from the 1980 Hayes and Flower model, and to elucidate their pivotal role in all phases of writing. Translation, in their revision, involves *text generation*, which happens internally as ideas are translated into language elements and held in the working memory, and thus they are independent of written production. Mental text generation takes advantage of cognitive language processes already in place, thereby facilitating this phase. *Transcription*, which takes language to paper, obligates the learning of novel skills, specifically spelling and handwriting, and, therefore, does not generalize easily from oral language ability. The transcription skills are considered to be low-level component writing processes (see Figure 4.1).

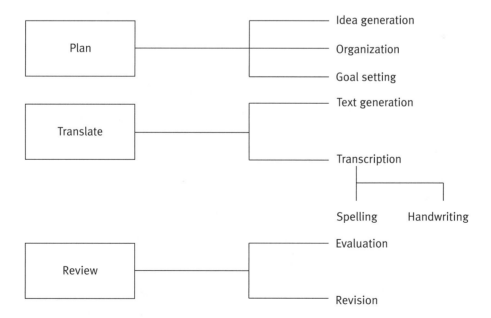

Figure 4.1. Recursive processes of writing.

A primary concern regarding process writing is the tendency to deemphasize or even eliminate the direct instruction of low-level skills, including spelling and handwriting, in favor of a stronger emphasis on the higher level cognitive elements (content over form, macro over micro). Handwriting and spelling, in the process writing or whole language approaches, may be expected to develop incidentally and informally (Graham, Harris, & Fink, 2000; Graham, Weintraub, & Berninger, 2001). Importantly, planning, translating, and reviewing do not always occur sequentially; rather, they interact recursively with each other as writing progresses.

The study of transcription skills, their relationship to each other, and their relationship to writing fluency and quality has vastly increased an awareness of the importance of handwriting in the writing process. The higher level cognitive processes, described by Hayes and Flower (1980), are now considered to be fundamental to *skilled* writing, whereas the lower level transcription skills are critical to the *acquisition* of writing and contribute heavily to individual differences in compositional fluency and quality in the primary grades. Similar to the consequences of any developmental constraint, difficulty in mastering handwriting and spelling is additionally implicated in children's discouragement, writing refusal, and ultimate failure in writing development (Abbott & Berninger, 1993). Conceptually, a good beginning point, then, is a discussion of handwriting and the linguistic and cognitive processes, handwriting and spelling as transcription partners, and then the neuromotor and visual-motor components of handwriting from the perspective of an OT.

HANDWRITING AND THE SHARED LINGUISTIC PROCESSES

Again, because handwriting is language by hand, the motoric output system and the internal linguistic and cognitive processes are closely allied in writing achievement. In addition, the linguistic processes variously underlie the three *modes* of output: manuscript writing, cursive handwriting and keyboarding. These three modes draw on both shared and unique components and differ in developmental characteristics from grade to grade in the primary years. Berninger and colleagues (2006) have contributed pivotally to this line of research. Their findings demonstrate, for example, that the ability to efficiently retrieve and produce the letters of the alphabet is foundational to printing skill and represents a primary constraint for the novice writer. Thus, RAN underlies manuscript *automaticity* in the first grade. Automaticity is not a simple measure of speed and accuracy, but it also reflects the freeing of cognitive resources via an internal and effective dispersion of conscious attention *away* from these formative processes. Higher level thinking, by its creative nature, does not become automatic and represents an understanding that heightens the need for the efficient processing of lower level skills.

The more automatically children retrieve the letter name from memory, the more automatically they will produce the letter on paper. If children struggle with RAN, it is likely that they will also have difficulty in printing automaticity. In addition to RAN, however, other linguistic processes also influence the speed and accuracy of printing. The first grader who struggles with RAN and orthographic coding is likely to struggle with printing *speed* because both linguistic components require rapid processing. The child who struggles with phonemic ability in the first grade is likely to have concurrent difficulty with printing accuracy (i.e., legibility of letter forms, correct ordering of the alphabet, and absence of reversals or inversions) because the letter–sound correspondence may be constrained. For example, if a child who wishes to print the word *dog* pairs grapheme to phoneme inaccurately, various inaccurate written combinations are possible (e.g., *bog, dok*). Conversely, the child may print a letter that correctly responds to an inaccurate analysis of the phoneme (e.g., *tall* instead of *call*).

In the third grade, according to Berninger and colleagues (2006), the underlying linguistic processes continue to allow predictions regarding manuscript accuracy and automaticity. Typing accuracy is additionally dependent on RAN and phonemic analysis. Moreover, phonemic abilities also play a role in cursive automaticity, illustrating the need for an efficient pairing of a letter's sound with its letter form counterpart in memory.

What does this mean to learning professionals as they work with children in real time? Handwriting, indeed, is influential in reading development for the typically developing child. Because the four functional language systems are both similar and unique, instruction should directly address the development of each, including handwriting as language by hand (Berninger et al., 2006). The teacher who best knows the child's linguistic abilities will contribute to an understanding of handwriting performance. The OT who evaluates handwriting dysfunction must be prepared to report not only the results of legibility and speed measures, but also to inform the team of the interplay between reported academic status and handwriting, as well as the likely educational impact of these findings.

SELF-REGULATION AS DEFINED IN THE WRITING PROCESS

Writing is a difficult and demanding goal-directed, multitask activity that requires high levels of executive control as the writer switches attention cyclically between levels in the writing process (Graham & Harris, 2000). The building blocks of self-regulation, from the cognitive perspective (different from the sensory perspective discussed in Chapter 5), include planning, monitoring, evaluating, and revising and are supported with a variety of strategies. Students with strong self-regulatory skills will set goals and plan composite steps, but will also seek information and assistance when needed. They will demonstrate organizational strategies, such as note taking or outlining, and may review and self-evaluate with effective rehearsal strategies, such as self-verbalization. They will structure the environment for best performance and budget time effectively. Selective and sustained attention support persistence with task. These characteristics of skilled writers account for a significant portion of the writing process and enhance overall performance. Struggling writers are less effective as self-regulators during composition, but they can be taught self-regulatory strategies to improve writing performance and confidence.

HANDWRITING AND SPELLING: TRANSCRIPTION PARTNERS

Handwriting automaticity (measured in practice by the number of legible letters a child can print within time constraints) and spelling covary significantly in the primary grades, which means that they may both limit and benefit each other and that they maintain stable relative positions so that predictions can be made about one skill by evaluating the developmental level of the other (Berninger et al., 2002). Together, the transcription skills contribute directly or indirectly to how much children write (compositional fluency) and how well they write it (compositional quality). In fact, these two components of writing account for two thirds of the individual differences in compositional fluency and one quarter of the individual differences in the quality of compositional content at the primary level (Graham, Berninger, Abbott, Abbott, & Whitaker, 1997).

Novice writers who are just learning spelling and handwriting, along with struggling writers who have not yet mastered transcription, are both constrained by the distribution of working memory to multiple demands because the writing processes constantly interrupt each other during the task. Transcription is costly to the short-term working memory of children in the primary grades and can be so difficult for some children that higher processes are minimized, creative solutions are suspended, and writing may be limited to less sophisticated styles, such as simple *retrieve-and-write* knowledge telling (Graham & Harris, 2000; McCutchen, 2000). It is, therefore, in the best interest of the young writing child to "indulge" the establishment of strong handwriting skills as a long-term benefit to writing achievement and to place significant and practical value on handwriting *automaticity* from the inception of the instructional process. When knowledge telling persists in older children, a collaborative approach will uncover clues about the child's difficulty in accessing and activating the higher level writing processes.

HANDWRITING IN THE SPELLING TASK

Several levels of central processing, as outlined by Rapp and Caramazza (1997), are activated before a word is written. Handwriting begins long before pencil hits paper. First, the word is retrieved from long-term memory storage of word meanings. If the word is simple or familiar, it is retrieved as a whole unit. If it is unfamiliar, nonsense, or complex, the *phonology–orthography conversion procedure* is activated. This means that the user is forced to sound it out and assign the appropriate corresponding letter. When this processing level is complete, the results are sent to short-term working memory and held there while further decisions are made and additional processing is begun. This holding store is conceptualized as a *graphemic buffer* and is independent of any mode of spelling expression. It is not invested in whether the person will spell orally or in writing, and, thus, it is an amodal, abstract mental representation. If the person decides to spell orally, he or she will begin one of the shared reading-writing processes—letter naming—and will pronounce each letter individually via the functional language-by-mouth system.

If required to produce a written product, the writer must first access the desired letter shape. Will he or she be writing in uppercase, lowercase, manuscript, cursive, italics, or calligraphy? These specific letter forms are called *allographs*, and they are assigned before the word is written. Once the allograph is accessed, it is further processed for its mechanical stroke features, including beginning points, anchor points (a term used in the drawing discussion in Chapter 3), and stroke direction and sequence. At this level, the writer has accessed a store of *graphic motor patterns*, which, again, are amodal representations that can be applied whether pencil on paper is used or the letter is formed with a handful of pebbles on the beach. When assisting children with the memory and recall of allographs and graphic motor patterns, letters can be formed in many ways, such as with clay or pipe cleaners. However, as discussed later in this chapter, the written product is best acquired and rehearsed by forming the letter strokes from their appropriate starting points and in their correct direction and sequence.

After accessing the graphic motor pattern, the writer is ready to execute the word motorically; activate the postural demands, pencil grasp, finger isolation, and dexterity; and subsequently be rewarded with a visible printed form. Because handwriting and spelling covary significantly at the primary level, the education team concerned with a child's handwriting will want to know whether the shared linguistic and cognitive processes are intact. When evaluating, I carefully read the assessment findings of the teachers for evidence of these skills and the findings of the school psychologist for evidence of memory and executive tendencies. If the child struggles with handwriting despite strong linguistic (including orthographic) abilities, and particularly if oral spelling is strong, it is important to look "farther down the line" for signs of confusion at the levels of the allographic or graphic motor pattern stores. These output precursors reflect the child's *internal* storage of form and stroke characteristics. Thus, prevention of later output problems should begin by ensuring efficient *recall* of the allograph and graphic motor pattern (see Figure 4.2).

Case mixing (lower- and uppercase confusion) can signal allographic instability despite effective instruction regarding the conventions of writing. A struggling student may well remember the rules, but he or she may not be able to call the appropriate allograph efficiently forward when actively engaged in a writing task. Often, as children focus on content, they may draw on the letter form that is most grounded in automaticity, which may lead them to mix upper with lowercase letters in mid-sentence. Here, children may benefit from the matching and sorting of letter forms, sorting of upper- and lowercase, or even haptic exercises that provide additional near-sense information regarding the differences in letter shape. Letter formation errors, however, may signal poorly stored graphic motor patterns. Assuming typical development of visual-motor ability and visual discrimination, this may be nothing more than an instructional issue, but it nevertheless highlights the importance of instructionally tending to the automaticity of letter

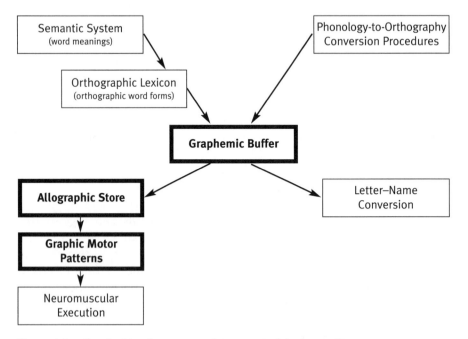

Figure 4.2. Handwriting (neuromuscular execution) in the spelling process.

production components and the early correction of flawed formations before habits are enduring and "unlearning" is required.

OTs often assess a student's visual-motor integration skills during the comprehensive evaluation. However, an understanding of the chain of processing active in *ortho-motor integration* should also be a significant consideration in the analysis of handwriting.

MOTOR PROFICIENCY AND HANDWRITING

Transcription skills (spelling and handwriting) constrain writing achievement, and shared linguistic processes constrain the efficiency of handwriting. What else uniquely constrains handwriting? Children's sensorimotor readiness is fundamental to their eventual success as writers under all task demands, whether they are writing for leisure or for standardized test taking. Recall the earlier appeal for *unencumbered* rehearsal as children experiment with movement and sort through less effective movement strategies to eventually uncover the most energy-efficient and cost-effective motor plan. During the motor learning process, wide performance fluctuations can be expected, and rehearsal of the novel physical task of handwriting is also substantially a cognitive task, just as it is an outward expression of the language-building brain. Early in handwriting development, young children also rely heavily on visual monitoring and fine motor *praxis* in the planning, sequencing, and execution of letter forms and letter strings. Praxis implies intentionality and direction toward a goal. Thus, the goal of letter formation and the goal of language production compete for cognitive and attentional resources at the word and sentence levels of composition.

This is not leading up to a call for the abandonment of the research-tested methodology of pairing reading and writing programs. It does, however, remind the education team of the need for motor rehearsal under less exacting academic task demands, which may mean, for example, an early and preferential focus on drama or drawing as literacy. It is an important consideration. The child whose motoric letter formation ability does not become automatic is at risk for long-term educational challenges or writing disability (Berninger, 2004).

Recently, even minor motor inefficiencies among young children without disabilities have proven to be associated with significant differences in handwriting proficiency. By using a computerized digitizing tablet, Rosenblum, Goldstand, and Parush (2006) have explored biomechanical ergonomic components during writing tasks. Children identified with poor handwriting consistently scored lower on all measures, and significant high correlations were found among ergonomic factors, with the exception of pencil grasp style. The quality of the written product was also negatively influenced, and, overall, Rosenblum's findings reflect the impact of biome-chanics and general motor efficiency on the transcription process of writing.

In other research, digital kinematic studies have shown significant differences in the movement strategies of good and poor writers, with poor writers showing cruder movement and more movement variability (*neuro-motor noise*) during the task (van Galen, Portier, Smits-Engelsman, & Schomaker, 1993). Studies of third and fourth graders have found that subtle increases in the variability of muscle activity in proximal (shoulder) and distal (hand) muscles is implicated in slower writing speed (Naider-Steinhart & Katz-Leurer, 2007). Thus, the economy of movement conserves physical expenditure and contributes to writing efficiency. Although teachers and OTs are unlikely to employ these high-tech methods in their team evaluations, the point is that the writing proficiency of young children is closely linked to effective motor support, which develops uniquely in trait and pace for each child in the primary grades.

Fine motor abilities, as evident in the language-by-hand motor output system, are influential in early applied pencil and paper activities. In the handwriting task, in-hand manipulation skills, particularly translation, have been found to predict legibility (i.e., formation, size, spacing, line orientation) in a near point copy assignment (Cornhill & Case-Smith, 1996). One specific measure of fine motor planning is rapid finger succession (i.e., touching each finger to thumb in turn), which proves to be one of the best predictors of handwriting performance in primary grades one through three (Berninger, 1999). This makes sense, considering the heavy influence of praxis (motor planning) on the ability to organize the movement sequences of handwriting. Also underlying motor proficiency are those sensory processing systems that monitor the touch and pressure of the pencil in hand and the direction and velocity of finger/hand movement, and that directly support postural readiness and head and/or vision stability through proprioceptive and vestibular sensory channels.

Orthographic coding and orthographic-motor integration also constrain handwriting, as described previously. In Berninger's research (1999), orthographic coding actually contributed more directly to handwriting development than the fine motor measures used in their study and was an excellent predictor of handwriting skill. Although this finding may appear to downplay the significance of a specific fine motor skill in the first, second, and third grades, Berninger observes that the relationship between handwriting and fine motor ability for 5-year-old children, although unexamined in their study, may prove to be more apparent. In my experience, this is certainly the case and constitutes one of the most important areas of shared knowledge in the development of a literacy program for children in kindergarten. In addition, more subtle relationships between motor and handwriting proficiencies have already been demonstrated and cannot be discounted throughout the primary level.

INFLUENCE OF GRASP STYLE AND HAND PREFERENCE ON HANDWRITING

Although many ergonomic factors do contribute to writing performance, research evidence of a strong impact of particular pencil grasp is uneven. To date, there is little documented influence of grasp style, whether tripod, lateral tripod, or other variation on writing legibility, speed, or endurance, although an expressed need for further research is consistent in the literature. (See Chapter 3 for a discussion of grasp styles.) At this time, it simply cannot be fully ruled in or out, nor can the long-term anatomical changes that may result from a less precise prehension be understood (Dennis & Swinth, 2001). In my experience, the more considerable variations can play into writing endurance and efficiency. Thus, it is my continuing recommendation to provide explicit instruction and monitoring for the dynamic tripod grasp in the primary grades with an expectation that some natural variation is common.

Differences in writing speed and legibility are not substantially apparent between left- and right-handed students (Ziviani & Elkins, 1986). Of course, for children with sensorimotor delays, the acquisition of both hand preference and an efficient grasp of the drawing or writing tool can be daunting and frustrating and will require support in the form of modifications or accommodations by the teacher and motor interventions by the OT.

VISUAL-MOTOR INTEGRATION

There is strong evidence that visual-motor integration is significantly related to a child's ability to legibly copy the letters of the alphabet in kindergarten (Daly, Kelley, & Krauss, 2003; Marr, Windsor, & Cermak, 2001; Weil & Cunningham Amundson, 1994). Although the excellent and commonly used *Beery-Buktenica Developmental Test of Visual-Motor Integration* (VMI) developed by Beery and Beery (2004) was designed neither as an evaluation of handwriting nor as a predictor of at-risk handwriting behavior, its strong psychometric properties make it a reliable and valid test of visual-motor integration skills. The research findings of Weil and Cunningham Amundson (1994) later replicated and supported by Daly and colleagues (2003) and Marr and colleagues (2001), confirm the use of the VMI to determine *readiness* for formal handwriting instruction among typically developing boys and girls. A significant difference in letter copying ability was found between children who were and were not able to copy the first nine forms on the VMI. In addition, letter copying ability increased as VMI scores improved. Mastery of the first nine forms on the assessment tool is therefore considered to be a printing prerequisite. These forms include:

Vertical line	I	Right oblique line	/
Horizontal line	—	Left oblique line	\
Circle	●	Oblique cross	X
Cross	+	Triangle	△
Square	■		

Because most children master these forms in the second half of the kindergarten year, these research teams find that most children should show readiness for formal manuscript instruction at that time. Thus, beginning explicit handwriting instruction in the latter half of the kindergarten year is considered developmentally appropriate practice. Beyond the readiness level, the relationship between handwriting and visual-motor integration is less consistent. The VMI, for example, although a valuable tool for determining printing readiness, is not a strong *predictor* of first-grade letter copy performance when administered to children in kindergarten (Marr & Cermak, 2002).

Consistent with other studies, Goyen and Duff (2005) found statistically significant differences in VMI scores between proficient and nonproficient handwriters in grades four through six. However, those with handwriting difficulty still scored within the normal range on the assessment tool. The researchers conclude that poor handwriting does not assume an underlying visual-motor disability. Conversely, poor visual-motor integration may be, but is not necessarily, associated with poor handwriting in the intermediate grades. Thus, the measurement of visual-motor integration skills and conclusions drawn from the results should be carefully weighed in the evaluation of handwriting, and detective work regarding the linguistic contributors to poor handwriting is a necessary part of the multidisciplinary evaluation process.

An additional and unexpected finding of Berninger's (1999) research is that visual-motor integration was found to be one of the best predictors of spelling performance! Children's knowledge and rapid encoding of letters has a considerable influence on handwriting, and their early treatment of spelling words as visual patterns significantly links spelling and visual-motor integration at the primary level.

THE DRAWING–WRITING LINK

Drawing is often undervalued, but it may be as constructive of early literacy as words on a page. Drawing units have a "grammar" of their own. They are ordered, symbolic, representational, communicative, and they convey meaning by visual image as surely as the meaning conveyed by letters or speech. Units of drawing, even though ordered in form and space, have polypotential to change, adapt, and "become" in intent. Writing is a closed system, constrained in the number of units (graphemes) that map the specific phonemic units of speech with little variation. Drawings are "read" by the child who is free to verbally embellish to his or her heart's content.

It is not uncommon for teachers to describe a child's inability to generate ideas. Often, teachers wonder about the student's fine motor ability and whether it may be a barrier in the writing process. How frustrating it must be for a child to expend minutes of unproductive time, only to become more discouraged as peers are busily putting words to paper around him. In the presence of typical fine and visual-motor ability, it can be a significant relief for such a child to develop a preliminary drawing plan. By activating visual-spatial in addition to language processing the child's ideas may readily flow, and the act of writing evolves from a reading of pictures and designs. Thus, the entire interhemispheric spatial and/or linguistic system is mobilized for action and outcome. Drawing and writing are both linguistic, and together they create a cross-modal approach to the communication of ideas (Sheridan, 1997).

☀ Maddy's Transition to Writing ☀

Maddy was a second grader who was thought to be distractible and poorly motivated. In the process of a comprehensive evaluation, I discovered her love of drawing and found that her visual-motor and spatial skills were above average for her age. Yet, writing was laborious for her, and the development of her writing plans was painstakingly slow. Every guiding question was met with "I don't know." If asked, "What would you like to write about," Maddy would answer, "I don't know." If asked, "What happens next," she would reply, "I don't know." This phrase was quickly becoming a form of writing refusal and threatening to become a permanent obstacle to educational performance in the writing process. I did not recommend OT services for Maddy, but rather suggested a liberal allowance of drawing as a prewriting strategy. Her teacher readily implemented the plan, initially requiring only a verbal retelling of her stories.

In a surprisingly short time, Maddy began to approach her assignments with heightened eagerness, and the ideas she so clearly and creatively communicated through drawing came progressively to life on the written page. A year later, I inquired about her and was delighted to hear of her great progress. By the middle of her third-grade year, Maddy was no longer relying on the drawing prewrite, but she did inform her teacher that she continued to develop a "mental drawing" before putting words to paper. Happily, over time, "I don't know" had faded.

As we have already discovered, drawing calls forward the same learning foundations of memory and executive function (i.e., planning, monitoring, and evaluating) and may focus the young child's attention and motivate more effectively than the written word. I am purposefully making a strong case for drawing. Drawing allows children to linger in the variability that is the hallmark of their age. It is a powerful organizer of thought and the sequence of idea and can later constitute a potent planning device in the prewriting process, much like an outline or other graphic organizer. Yet, through the K–3 educational level, its use declines, and drawing tends to become the afterthought of writing, used primarily for illustrating text. One study found that first graders included drawings in 84% of their written tasks. By third grade, the percentage had fallen to less than 50% (Colello, 2001).

The drawing and writing systems are notational relatives, and numerous studies have investigated the relationship between the two. Are the systems distinct, or does one gradually emerge from the other? It appears that the answer is "yes" to both possibilities depending on the research question.

When referring to drawing and writing as areas of *domain-specific knowledge* (what children know about objects versus what they know about words), some findings suggest that the two systems are distinct (Brenneman, Massey, Machado, & Gelman, 1996; Landsmann & Karmiloff-Smith, 1992). Children as young as 3 years, for example, will produce pseudowriting that has the distinct characteristics of writing rather than those of drawing. Pseudowriting is produced with linearity, left–right directionality, discrete graphic units, short strokes, and regular spaces. Drawing employs outlines; filled-in surfaces; and more liberal, less constrained use of the spatial field. When asked to "write" the word *cow*, the action plan and the product will look very different than those resulting in a *picture* of the animal. Thus, young children already seem to know that a drawing must look like its referent, whereas writing does not. Even the child's affect will reflect the difference and reveal more thinking behavior during pretend writing (Brenneman et al., 1996). Although environmental models and childish mimicry certainly play a role in the graphic and behavioral differentiation of the two systems, domain-specific knowledge lends a strong and early influence.

On the contrary, Adi-Japha and Freeman (2001) have researched the relationship from a *kinematic* perspective, looking specifically at the characteristics of arm and hand motion during writing and drawing tasks, and the authors reached a different conclusion. Their inspiration was derived from medical findings in which adults with neurological impairment can lose their drawing ability while retaining the ability to write (and vice versa), which suggests two distinct neural systems. The additional observation that pretend writing produces a writing-like product also prompts their investigation.

Specific movement characteristics, however, suggest a single early system that differentiates over time. At age 4, there is no difference in evident motion patterns between drawing and writing, despite differences in the appearance of the product. After age 6, kinematic control begins to show more efficiency during the writing task. Drawing will become relatively slower and less fluent, and the distinction is retained into adulthood. An experiment, similar to a task in the Adi-Japha (2001) study, involves the following:

1. Write the words *noon, soon,* and *moon.*

2. Draw a box that represents a birdhouse.

3. Place six aligned entry holes on your drawing.

Even though the shapes are exactly the same, it is likely that the o's in the words were produced more quickly and fluently than the entrances on the birdhouse. Writing and drawing have differentiated.

The writing-specific system gradually emerges from an undifferentiated drawing system that the 4-year-old uses to both produce pictures and to "draw" pretend print. Whereas motion patterns begin to differentiate at 6 years, the child at this transitional age works actively to suppress interference from the drawing system. Vocabulary tasks, such as writing a word after viewing its pictorial image, require cognitive sorting and drawing suppression and may actually retard writing automaticity, according to the researchers. The need to suppress the drawing system declines as the two systems differentiate and as writing increases in automaticity.

A blended conclusion might well consider both research perspectives. Both drawing and writing are linguistic in the intent to communicate idea. Young children seem to distinguish between their *knowledge* of the two notational systems; however, motion studies support the gradual *kinematic* emergence of writing from drawing. Although many authors and educators endorse the blending of writing and drawing as early as kindergarten (e.g., in drawing and labeling), conflict in differentiating the two systems graphically may suggest the need for patience in the formal introduction of handwriting and a greater reliance on drawing as literacy in the kindergarten year.

READY FOR INSTRUCTION:
WHERE DO WE START?

At this point, evidence of many shared processes in the reading–writing link is eminently clear, and simultaneous instruction of both literacy components is becoming a familiar best practice. The nagging remaining question is one of timing. When kindergartners engage in prompted writing exercises before they have been formally introduced to all letter formations, they often struggle with *invented handwriting* as well as invented spelling. Whereas invented spellings typically self-correct as phonological and orthographic coding skills mature, poor letter formations are more likely to become stable but inefficient graphic productions. In the long run, time devoted to the stabilization of accurate allographs and graphic motor patterns and their efficient retrieval from long-term memory will be a valuable investment in the future of writing performance. A more holistic systems approach and a careful vetting of the student–environment–task interplay will inspire a preemptive model at the level of core instruction.

It is clear that many children are simply not prepared for early handwriting instruction, as was learned in previous discussions of visual-motor integration and the recognition of the developmental ranges at the primary level. The proliferation of remedial strategies and special education referrals for handwriting difficulty is testament to this, in my opinion. I would much prefer that education teams take an unhurried and preventive approach to handwriting for young learners. I know this raises questions. What about the children who are ready? How do we pedagogically address the research-based reading–writing link? How do we address literacy skills if we postpone formal handwriting instruction? I am convinced that the more education teams collaborate on these issues with team members, parents, preschool teachers, and policymakers, the more creatively they will develop comprehensive best practice solutions, prevent later writing deficiencies, and reduce the need for remedial interventions. The mutual goal, after all, is a strong literacy foundation that serves all children unfailingly as academic demands increase and that is built (as research confirms) on the mastery and automaticity of the lower level processes.

Teachers have many questions about the instruction of handwriting for young children. Rightfully so. There are many programs, each with its preferred manuscript and cursive styles and each with its own procedures and presentation sequences. The following sections establish some basic priorities regarding the *process* of instruction.

Most Efficient Instruction at the Most Effective Time

The best time to begin formal handwriting instruction is in the latter half of the kindergarten year. In addition, it should be taught for automaticity through a carefully designed instructional and rehearsal process. Once children are ready, the following steps of group instruction and guided practice are quite simple and incorporate several principles of motor control, multi-modal learning, and procedural memory enhancement. I have found finger tracing to be a highly effective tactile and kinesthetic strategy in facilitating the stability of graphic motor patterns and often use this sequence to teach even the basic shapes (i.e., circle, square, and triangle) to children with developmental delays. Once a writing tool is placed in the hand, there is a physical barrier between body and paper, and tactile-proprioceptive cues are less direct.

A method I call the *five-step handwriting process* (described step by step in this section) is appropriate for new learning and is particularly effective as targeted intervention for children who struggle with handwriting development. It can be used for small or whole class groups. Before beginning the process, children should be seated at a table or desk directly facing the teacher. Facing different directions will complicate the task perceptually and will risk an inefficient path to the accurate graphic motor pattern. The teacher should have large bold model letters *with numbered arrows* (the size depends on the size of the group). The children should have smaller but sturdy models of each letter (approximately 4 inches tall on heavy paper, cardstock, or laminated sheets) and paper and pencil. The use of numbered arrows facilitates the automatization of stroke direction and sequence and serves as a bridge to memory (Berninger et al., 1997). Some initial introduction to their use will be helpful to the children.

Prior to beginning, experiment with paper. Whether it is lined or unlined should not significantly influence the child's product during this early acquisition phase. Some children may do better with just a baseline; blank or lined primary papers will be more effective for others. My only caution is that wide rule notebook paper, which is used for many kindergarten

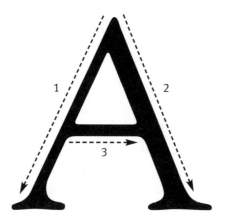

writing journals, is the least desirable choice for beginners. Although it is readily available for parents as a purchased school item, it provides ill-defined visual support for children who are just learning the spatial requirements of handwriting.

The teacher then chooses three target letters for the week's lesson. Those uppercase letters with matching motor patterns (Cc, Oo, Ss) require less time spent on formation, but definite attention to spatial orientation when using lined paper. (*Note:* for the following procedure, be sure to instruct children to use their *worker hand* for all finger tracing.) The following list delineates the five-step handwriting process.

1. Model: Teacher *names* target letter while *finger tracing* the large model in correct stroke sequence. Avoid using action or locative words to describe the movements (e.g., "go down," "across"). Remember that the motor centers of children's brains are firing while they are watching. Any verbalizations, other than the name of the letter, are distracting and unnecessary. This, however, is obviously modified with tactile support and verbal strategies for the child with some visual impairment.

2. Air Writing: Teacher demonstrates by *finger tracing* a second time. Children imitate by naming the letter and finger writing *in the air* (pretending to trace over the teacher's formation from a distance). This is an important step that allows the teacher to quickly catch formation errors in the group. Immediately correct the errors.

3. Finger Tracing: Teacher demonstrates again (third time), then children name the letter and *finger trace* their own smaller arrowed letter model three times. (Finger tracing is used variably in instructional process. See, e.g., Graham et al., 2000.)

4. Memory Writing: Children *turn their model over* and *use pencil or crayon and paper* to produce the letter immediately and quietly *from memory* three times. Producing from memory is significant in stabilizing the graphic motor pattern and is often missing from beginning handwriting instruction (Berninger et al., 1997). Three rehearsals aid procedural memory and also allow the teacher time to scan the classroom for children struggling with the process.

5. Rehearsal: During the course of a 15-minute instructional session, children are presented in *random rotating order* the three target letters for the week.

Guided Rehearsal During Brief Supervised Lessons

Five- to ten-minute sessions several times throughout the week in addition to the initial five-step introduction will provide necessary practice while children are learning. Once children are familiar with the process, they may be excited and able to practice steps 3 and 4 on their own and can retrieve their models and materials for independent work. If so, be sure to check in occasionally to ensure correct letter formation as the child works, remembering that the product on a completed page can belie an ineffectual production process. First-grade review should follow the same steps initially.

It is now widely agreed that explicit instruction and practice are necessary for fluency of the transcription processes. Regarding handwriting, research has focused on two strands of inquiry. First, do children without disabilities benefit more from a rehearsal of the underlying sensorimotor components of the task (i.e., in-hand manipulation, visual-motor integration, visual perception, and kinesthesia) or from a direct rehearsal of letter formation and compositional application? Denton, Cope, and Moser (2006) found that therapeutic practice, or direct rehearsal, is the more effective intervention for children who struggle with handwriting performance. This is consistent with my own finding that explicit practice of the precise motor pattern facilitates stabilization in memory. Supplementary activities such as forming letters with clay or pipe cleaners are wonderful fine motor alternatives for awareness of the allograph. Facilitation of the stability of the graphic motor pattern, however, will require rehearsal of the exact stroke formation and sequence, which can be accomplished creatively and multimodally by writing in clay or sand. Of course, the OT will incorporate additional interventions targeted to underlying processes for children with sensorimotor disabilities.

The second strand of inquiry is whether blocked practice is more effective than random practice. Ste-Marie, Clark, Findlay, and Latimer (2004) specifically examined the effects of varying practice schedules on handwriting and found that a random schedule is more effective for the acquisition, retention, and transfer of letter formations. Blocked practice involves the repetition of a single letter over numerous trials (e.g., XXXX..., YYYY..., ZZZZ...). Random practice, however, offers a mixed presentation of target letters (e.g., XYXZZYX...). In this study, the more effortful cognitive processing required for the random practice schedule resulted in greater permanence and adaptability of learning. Children were better able to retain the letter formations over time and could more easily apply their knowledge at the word level. Although research findings are variable in the literature, the results of Ste-Marie et al. (2004) are consistent with principles of motor learning. Because consolidation of motor memories only begins *after* practice stops (Sousa, 2001), several guided weekly rehearsals are critical for retention. Given the research findings on practice, the five-step handwriting process incorporates a random practice schedule during the acquisition phase of instruction. Teachers will find additional and creative ways to facilitate the critical need for handwriting automaticity (some of which are addressed in Chapter 6).

Furthermore, I am not personally invested in one particular published handwriting curriculum over another, but rather in the effort toward the timing of instruction based on visual-motor readiness, the recruitment of sensory amplification for motor learning, the critical necessity of bridging to memory, and the most efficient rehearsal pattern for automaticity. Handwriting instruction both precedes and extends beyond the introduction of letter formation and is a *process* for both teacher and learner.

Additional Tips and Cautions

Handwriting Style: Vertical or Slanted?

The preference my colleagues and I have for a vertical manuscript is supported by research, despite past claims of the superiority of a slanted style (Graham, 1993/1994; Graham, Weintraub, & Berninger, 1998; Kuhl, 1994). In the 1980s, the slanted D'Nealian alphabet was adopted by major scholastic publishers and many local school districts after persuasive arguments concerning the ease of transition to cursive script, the rhythm and speed of more continuous strokes, the moderation of reversals, and the ease of formation for children with disabilities (see www.dnealian.com). My own experience tells of OTs and teachers who are convinced otherwise. Novice printers may fail to orient their letters on a slant, and the extra strokes and tails add to the motor planning challenge of task demand. There is no convincing research evidence for a more effective cursive transition or for the superiority of a continuous stroke formation (Graham, 1993/1994). Given the discussions of the reading–writing link and the need for established allographs (letter forms) in long-term memory, the visual consistency between words that are read and words that are written would be a natural priority for young children. Having said this, many school districts who have already adopted the D'Nealian alphabet may have limited financial resources for an immediate change of literacy programs. It is, therefore, incumbent on the education team to ensure a well conceived process-oriented method for the introduction of handwriting, which will be central to the prevention of learning barriers in writing achievement.

Which Comes First? Upper- or Lowercase?

From a visual-motor perspective, uppercase letters are easier for young children because they all start at the top, and each is spatially oriented from headline to baseline. However, it is not practical to wait on the presentation of the more frequently used lowercase letters, and a combined approach should not create confusion if formal and systematic instruction awaits readiness later in the kindergarten year. Tending to automaticity in the recall and production of the appropriate allograph will be preventive regarding case sensitivity and line orientation as children enter compositional writing.

Letter Sequence: Alphabetic or Kinesthetic?

Depending on teacher preference and whether a published handwriting program is used, there is significant variation in the sequence of letter introduction. A theme-oriented approach is used by some (e.g., A for apple week), whereas others recommend a kinesthetic approach (a term often interchangeable with proprioception) that groups letters by common stroke starting points or directions. Based on research of the acquisition of motor skills and the development of long-term memory, however, there is equally convincing evidence for the grouping of letters that have very *different* allographic forms and/or graphic motor patterns. It is common to teach similar spelling patterns or concepts together. However, we also know that retention can be compromised when similarities outweigh the differences or critical attributes in new information (Sousa, 2001) (e.g., do you recall the difference between stalactites and stalagmites?). Motor research reveals similar challenges to retention when skills with very similar motor patterns are taught together. Again, the handwriting process is most crucial to acquisition and retention. Beyond the process, I would suggest that teachers avoid grouping commonly confused or reversed letters together in the same instructional session (e.g., *b, d, p, q*), and I would also suggest avoiding the grouping of very similar motor patterns (e.g., *m/n, w/v*). In addition, the prioritization of vowels and commonly used letters may facilitate the application to the writing process at the word level.

Provide Extra Practice for Difficult Letters

From first through third grades, five lowercase formations accounted for the majority of legibility errors in the research of Graham et al. (2001). They are: *q, z, u, j,* and *k*. Lowercase g, n, and y created additional difficulty for first graders. Watch for the most common formation errors, which include the addition of *extra* strokes (e.g., concentric circular strokes) and poor proportion of parts.

Pencil Tracing and Dot-to-Dot

I do not recommend pencil tracing or dot-to-dot for the instruction of letter formation. In general, pencil tracing (over forms without arrow cues) as the primary form of acquisition or rehearsal is a simple visual-motor exercise that significantly reduces the cognitive processing and memory components of learning and impedes the establishment of the graphic motor pattern. I find that dot-to-dot letters are visually busy and may direct cognitive resources toward dot connection, rather than the processing and memory storage of motor pattern sequences. When a fifth-grade boy with developmental delays transferred into one of my schools, a change in task demand afforded him the acquisition of an elusive functional skill. Despite years of practice, he had not yet learned to print his first name, and solid letter tracing was the recommended method on his individualized education program (IEP). After several unsuccessful days of trial, we began to use the five-step handwriting process, and he was independently and correctly printing his name within 2 weeks.

How to Teach Letter and Word Spacing

This visual-spatial concept tends to be closely linked to orthographic awareness in young or struggling writers. When the chunking of letters in words is not understood, the chunking of letters on the page will not be a priority. When children struggle with spelling, cognitive resources are directed away from the spatial components of handwriting, and legibility can suffer. I use analogies for spacing. For young children, I sometimes talk about families, houses, and yards. The letters of a word are members of the same family and live in the same house, and so they live close together. Between each house is a big back yard. This analogy is easily adapted to towns and roads, tables in the classroom, or other spatial concepts in sensitivity to the circumstances of the child. For children who continue to struggle, try also using 1/2-inch graph paper. Print a model with one letter per space and two or three spaces between words. For older children, I often use a keyboarding analogy to have the student mentally "hit the space bar" between words. However, the most important strategy for the new learner is *to over space the words in the teacher's visual models*. If a computerized system is used, place several spaces between words on the white board or screen. Be attentive to the very poor spacing model that is offered on many published worksheets and avoid their use. Online resources with lined paper samples can be accessed to create a bank of teacher-made worksheets that are designed with relevant content and overspaced wording.

Legibility versus "Readability"

When collaborating on the appearance of a student's finished product, it often becomes clear that legibility is a secondary issue. Misspelled words, syntactical errors, and omitted letters or words can all have an impact on the readability of the work, whereas letter and word legibility are within typical limits. Yet, the initial concern over messy handwriting may presume poor visual-motor or spatial awareness.

Handwriting Speed

Given the opportunity to use their most efficient personal writing mode (i.e., manuscript, cursive, or mixed style) and assuming that linguistic processes are intact, children's handwriting speed increases by spurts and plateaus from first grade, but by roughly 10 letters per minute until students begin to approximate adult speed in ninth grade (Graham, Berninger, Weintraub, & Schafer, 1998). Girls are typically faster than boys, and left handers may be slowed slightly by their tendency to adjust the paper position more frequently. There is little association between handwriting speed and legibility, although children can adjust their speed when asked in order to focus on neatness. Remember that underlying linguistic processes may be at work in both handwriting speed and legibility and should be carefully screened when writing output does not meet grade level or teacher expectations. Finally, it is helpful to take a larger overview of handwriting speed and legibility in the classroom, as teachers do not typically measure writing speed. Are students' products legible (and readable) to themselves and others? Do they maintain a pace commensurate with the linguistic and cognitive capacities of *their own* written expression ability? If not, targeted interventions or evaluation for specially designed instruction may be warranted.

Handwriting Embedded

Once readiness is determined and formal handwriting instruction is under way, reading and writing can be actively linked in tasks that embed handwriting in the writing process as long as initial rehearsal is provided during instruction. Children may actually be more motivated to further practice handwriting when their efforts produce simple words *with learned letters* rather than long strings of letters, and their creative thinking as authors is inspired. As discussed previously, letter legibility is not well served by overpractice of long letter strings (blocked practice) because fatigue and disinterest may influence successive trials until the last letter produced and remembered is also the most poorly formed.

How, then, can the need for handwriting automaticity through unencumbered rehearsal be reconciled with the understanding that the acquisition of an alphabetic writing system appears to facilitate phonemic awareness? A balance of student–environment–task demand will require careful management in ensuring the automaticity of transcription skills as higher level academic expectations are introduced. Many more pencilless strategies (which are discussed in Chapter 6) will creatively stabilize both allograph and graphic motor pattern and constitute a preventive approach to performance barriers.

A WORD ABOUT CURSIVE AND KEYBOARDING

I have been approached many times about the elimination of cursive handwriting instruction. Once children reach the secondary level, it is true that the cursive style is often no longer required and that many students use a word processing mode for final drafts. The only answer to the question of cursive will come through a collaborative approach in the educational community. What we do know is that cursive handwriting is actually not faster than manuscript (assuming similar instruction and rehearsal), and that there is no difference in either legibility or speed between the two handwriting modes for children without disabilities (Graham, Berninger et al., 1998). For children who struggle, however, cursive handwriting can naturally release attentional resources otherwise allocated to letter and word spacing, and cursive writing is often the recommended mode for children with specific learning disabilities. By the fourth grade, children's writing styles have typically stabilized, and the fastest style is often a manuscript-cursive combination. It is best to allow students to develop a natural and personal style that will serve their own needs in the writing process. Regarding the instructional method of cursive handwriting, the tactile-kinesthetic finger tracing strategy is generally no longer necessary for typically developing children, and a visual demonstration and model with direct student trial will most likely suffice for students who participate at the level of core instruction.

The recommendation of word processing as an alternative to handwriting at the level of targeted intervention takes into consideration elements of the entire writing process. The various modes of writing (i.e., manuscript, cursive, and keyboarding) share common underlying processes, but also rely on unique processes that may variously influence performance in the three modes (Berninger et al., 2006). The elimination of handwriting mechanics, therefore, may not circumvent all problem areas for the writer who will bring his or her own neuromotor and linguistic abilities to the keyboard. There is no doubt that computer use is an important instructional element of 21st century education and that assistive technology in the form of spell check, talking word processing, word prediction, and organizational software is invaluable to children who struggle with the lower and higher level processes of writing. However, handwriting and keyboarding do not translate straight across, and a decision to replace handwriting is best made by the education team who can consider all student factors, environmental components, and task demands within the collaborative prevention model.

PLANNING FOR SUCCESS

There are many excellent resources for methodologies in the remediation of handwriting dysfunction. The OT can bring a wealth of wonderful ideas to the classroom. To supplement the foundational principles of this chapter, this section reviews a starter kit of strategies with additional focus on preparation and prevention.

- Addressing sensory and attentional needs: Consider a study carrel for the student who is sensitive to environmental distraction; alert the underresponsive child (see Chapter 5) with a bright placemat or place tactile surfaces (e.g., sandpaper, fine needlepoint grid) under drawing or writing work; encourage alternative positioning (e.g., on the floor) for postural stability in young children; use drawing as a prewrite; schedule extended writing work after PE or recess; take plenty of movement breaks.

- Developing motor proficiency: Begin a handwriting lesson with isometric arm and hand exercises to wake up the motor output system. Push hands firmly together, do *finger pushups* with hands together, or against the table. Do chair pushups by raising the body off the seat surface and pushing with hands on the edge of the chair; offer dynamic seating options to the underresponsive or sensory-seeking child; have many fine motor and manipulative play options in the classroom; post graffiti paper on the wall to encourage drawing on a vertical surface; always have short crayons available for children with immature prehension; embed movement generously in all learning!

- Preventing extended reversals (common through age 7): Play haptic games with letters; play air-writing games with pre-letter shapes using *large* arm movements; accompany movement directions with silly vocal sounds instead of locative terms (always using the same sound for the same direction). Because it directly engages the near senses of the body, finger tracing in the five-step handwriting process should strongly cue directionality in letter formation.

- Motivating neat handwriting: Timely and explicit handwriting instruction and early priority on automaticity through effective instructional process and rehearsal will naturally prevent much of the frustration and discouragement that can result in joyless writing or writing refusal. Once writing, however, not all children place a high priority on neatness for a variety of reasons. For older students, assign 10-minute fluency exercises by having them copy out of a favorite book. Have them concentrate on only one or two target problems for each exercise (e.g., spacing, a specific letter formation, line orientation). Try using teacher–student contracts that are turned in with the final draft and that focus the child's attention on the production and/or correction of the targeted areas of need (see Figure 4.3). Consider handwriting groups (similar to reading groups) for spot checks and mini lessons.

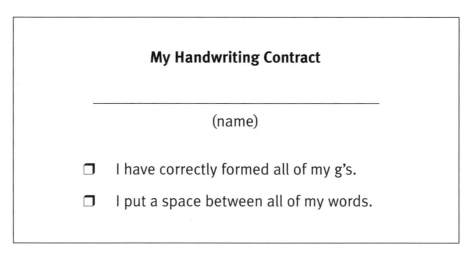

Figure 4.3. Teacher–student contract to encourage handwriting neatness.

- Accommodating left handers: Assist with paper position by slanting the paper to the right (corner at belly); place a slanted tape line on the desk as a reminder; remember that when left-handed children write, they may effectively eliminate their visual cues for spacing and will subsequently challenge their short-term memory for spelling by covering the previously printed letters with their hand and arm. Design a set of spelling lists for left handers that places the words on the right edge of the page so that the model is clearly visible when copying for practice.

☀ Doing the Detective Work: Two Case Studies ☀

Ben and Nadya represent the discovery process in uncovering the possible barriers to fluent and legible handwriting, and the variables of remediation. Ben is a sixth grade student, whose handwriting has always been nearly undecipherable, and during his fifth grade year he was issued a portable word processor and math software to support academic output. His medical diagnosis places him on the autism spectrum, and he is considered "twice exceptional," having cognitive abilities in the superior range. Ben is enrolled in the gifted program and will soon transition to the secondary level. Figure 4.4 demonstrates two of Ben's handwriting samples, both taken within 5 minutes during the same OT session. The first represents his typical performance, difficult even for Ben to reread himself. The second follows the introduction of a single modification. What might be the student factors, environmental components, and task demands that contribute to such a striking difference in performance?

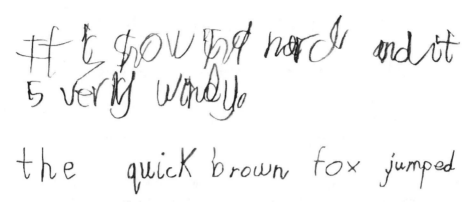

Figure 4.4. Change in handwriting performance following simple modification of writing tool.

Working from central to peripheral processes during the evaluation, it is determined that Ben's phonemic and orthographic abilities are strong and supportive, and do not contribute to his handwriting dysfunction. A visual inspection of the legible sample discloses a predominantly effective use of case, along with consistent and accurate letter forms. Ben's allographic store is intact and stable. Observations of writing in progress determine that Ben is additionally forming his letter strokes in correct directions and sequences, reflecting an efficient memory store of graphic motor patterns.

Having determined the stability of the central processes for this talented young man, further detective work is required to discover the barrier to motor execution during handwriting itself. While Ben's motor abilities are in the low-average range, an assessment of sensory processing reveals that the greatest obstacle lies in his significant sensitivity to touch. As he writes, it appears as though he is anxious to throw the pencil out of his hand after every stroke.

The week following this revealing observation and assessment, Ben was presented with several fabric samples and asked to choose the texture that was most comfortable for him – a soft lightweight fleece. After simply wrapping the pencil with the fleece and eliminating the tactile performance barrier, the clarity of Ben's handwriting is immediately and astoundingly enhanced. Although Ben will require intensive fluency practice with his new and somewhat slower production, his class work is becoming increasingly legible, and his pride increasingly evident.

Nadya is a 2nd-grader, also referred for evaluation of "messy handwriting." In her case the discovery of performance barriers proceeded from peripheral to central abilities. Figure 4.5 demonstrates Nadya's production

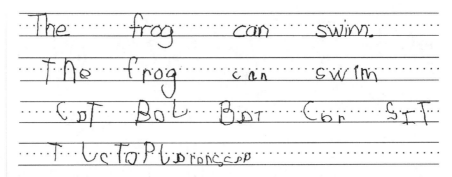

Figure 4.5. Second-grade handwriting sample illustrating how linguistic demands increasingly overwhelm legibility during copy, dictation, and composition.

under the 3 variable task demands of near-point copy, dictation, and composition. Assessment of visual-motor skills reveals her average range performance in this domain, and the copy task reflects age-appropriate letter formation, line orientation, and letter/word spacing. It becomes obvious, however, that the increasing linguistic demands of dictation and composition progressively tax Nadya's fragile allographic and graphic motor pattern stores. Letter reversals emerge, letter formation declines, and spatial consistency disappears.

For Nadya, three conclusions generate the remediation plan. First, multidisciplinary evaluation reveals that Nadya is struggling with central phonemic and orthographic skills and is quickly becoming disenchanted with the writing process. Second, it is determined that the lower level transcription processes of handwriting production are not sufficiently stable or automatic, and do not hold up under increasingly rigorous task demand, despite average motor proficiency. Third, it is concluded that Nadya's attempt to accommodate poor handwriting automaticity results in an inefficient allocation of cognitive and memory resources, creating a significant barrier to idea generation and quality of content during compositional writing.

Intervention for Nadya, after consideration of assessment results, includes remediation of central linguistic processes, letter formation review using the finger-tracing method of the five step handwriting process, unencumbered rehearsal of letter formation, drawing prewrites to enhance the organization of thoughts and the sequence of ideas, and a gradual embedding of handwriting in simple word production during compositional tasks.

The finding of average range visual-motor skills for both of these students did not conclude the detective work to uncover the primary handwriting barriers and to suggest the most precise intervention strategies. While both case studies reflect the multiple components of handwriting performance, Nadya's clearly demonstrates the linguistic nature of the task and the highly integrated path of evaluation and targeted remediation.

FINAL THOUGHTS:
THE PREVENTION FRAME OF MIND

The focus of this chapter has not been devoted primarily to handwriting hints and strategies, but rather to the conceptual link between teacher and OT expertise in addressing the broad elements of writing performance. The principal aim is to remind the education team, including teachers and OTs, about the position of handwriting in the writing process and to ensure teachers of their irrefutable role in the evaluation of handwriting. The chapter also highlights the need for a *preventive,* rather than a remedial, approach to handwriting, with four lines of focus. First is an understanding of the linguistic nature of handwriting and its relationship to other linguistic processes. Second is the development of policies addressing the most effective timing of explicit handwriting instruction, along with a research-based instructional process. Third is an early prioritization of the automaticity of handwriting skills, which may mean a slight rethinking of the implementation of the reading–writing link and a higher priority on the internal stability of allographic and graphic motor pattern stores prior to extensive pencil use. Fourth is the early focus on creative and collaborative literacy strategies that include "writing *without* writing" activities and a reliance on drama, play, or drawing-as-literacy prior to the inception of formal handwriting instruction in kindergarten, as well as the continuing support of idea generation and planning in the writing process through the primary grades.

I am frequently reminded of the need for early automaticity and cannot underscore it strongly enough. Multiple referrals for OT evaluation throughout a single child's primary years are not uncommon when handwriting is poorly legible. Yet, motor proficiency may be well within the average range. The lesson regarding the reading–writing link and the connection between handwriting and writing process is striking. The automaticity of lower level transcription skills is critical for all students as a foundation for compositional fluency and quality. However, when a young child struggles with early reading precursors, with linguistic processes such as phonemic awareness, RAN, or orthographic coding, a red flag should surely be raised. Freedom to devote attentional and memory resources to higher level thinking is the goal. Awaiting keyboarding fluency is not a tenable solution for the child who is rapidly losing the motivation to express ideas in print.

Indeed, the collaborative model based on an exploration of the student–environment–task interplay is applied to curriculum design, core instruction, targeted intervention, and progress monitoring as a critical element in the deterrence of preventable dysfunction through an integration of expertise for this heavily integrated task. It is facilitated by a collective understanding of student factors in the areas of neurodevelopmental, linguistic, and cognitive abilities and of the implications of task demand as novel skills are rehearsed for automaticity.

My observations and those of many of my colleagues are of concern for the school-related stress factors affecting young children, particularly with regard to the developmental manageability of the increasing writing expectations at the primary level. Such preeminence is placed on writing achievement that wisdom in the methods of instruction and patience in the timing are necessary to engage all children successfully and happily as authors of the stories they weave and communicators of the solutions they dream.

5

Seven Senses in School

Teachers can perform a magnificent feat. They can manage the random chatter of 30 active classmates and still focus the discussion toward a desired and meaningful educational outcome. This is no small achievement. Organization is required, and strategies must be developed to increase attention to the important elements of a task. The focused work of small groups can often bring greater clarity to a project, benefiting the efficiency of the academic product as a whole and achieving the desired goal. The raw materials of the classroom are recruited, organized, integrated, and put to purposeful use, and children learn.

Now imagine having 100 *billion* students whose conversational connections number in the *trillions*. Organization is impossible, and even the most patient of teachers would understandably be frazzled. Attention and focus? Forget it. Noise level? Earsplitting. Will consensus be reached on the goal? Not a chance. Yet, organization of billions of connections is what the central nervous system (CNS) does effectively every moment of every day.

The 100 billion "students" are neurons in the brain—nerve cells designed specifically to communicate with each other over space and time—and the brain is the only organ in the body whose cells have this capacity to exchange information (LeDoux, 2002). Over the course of a few pages, it is impossible to address every level and every mechanism by which the CNS integrates sensation with sensation, sensation with movement, and sensation with cognition toward a successful behavioral response. This chapter touches on only a few of these astounding neural strategies while reviewing the role of sensory processing in the balance of student factors, environmental components, and task demands in school.

ORGANIZATIONAL STRATEGIES OF THE BRAIN

Your body is tuned to receive. Receptors in the skin harvest touch, temperature, pain, and pressure. Receptors in your muscles and joints collect evidence—*proprioception*—of the active movement and position of your body in space relative to the force of gravity. Proprioception is generally a subconscious sense; therefore, we are unaware of its function or its dysfunction (Melillo & Leisman, 2004). The feedback provided by proprioception informs the brain of the sensations of movement and cues the adjustment of the body for movement and balance. The inner ear manages specialized proprioception through the *vestibular* apparatus in the semicircular canals, which collect information about the movement of the head in space, as well as its movement in relation to the body. Vestibular sensation adds to the fine tuning of posture and is important in stabilizing the visual field (Goldberg & Hudspeth, 2000; Jones, 2000). Thousands of bits of various sensations enter the system at a given moment, and, if not organized and prioritized, they would be nothing more than random sensory "chatter" (LeDoux, 2002).

Humans are consciously aware of only a small portion of this great volume of sensation, but none of it goes to waste. As it enters the brain from all parts of the body and the environment, much of it is sent to higher cortical centers in two ways. Some travels to special centers in the cerebral cortex, each of which is designed to process *modality-specific* information (e.g., for vision or hearing). Other sensations are sent nonspecifically or diffusely throughout the cortex and serve an important pacemaker-type function by providing constant rhythmic stimulation to maintain a baseline level of arousal or alertness (Melillo & Leisman, 2004). Neither pathway is more important than the other. In fact, without baseline arousal, we would not be alert enough to make sense of discrete messages of sound, vision, or touch. Proprioception from the spinal postural muscles, which respond to gravitational forces, provides the most constant stream of subconscious sensation to feed the arousal needs of the wakeful brain, making the movement of the body a powerful partner in learning readiness. When baseline information decreases, we may become drowsy, hopefully at the right time of day.

The neuron itself is designed to organize information. These unique cells are built to receive electrical messages through tiny projections around the cell body and then to send the message along to other neurons through a longer nerve fiber or axon (Gertz, 2007). With so many sensory messages coming in at one time, how do we avoid succumbing to information overload? The neuron has it covered. An electrical message is activated and passed along only when the sensory stimulation is strong enough, frequent enough, intense enough, or arrives simultaneously from multiple neuron senders. Otherwise the receiving neuron is designed to stay quiet. The axon can branch, which allows a single neuron to pass its signal on to several others and increase the breadth of the message. Conversely, the cell body of a single neuron can also *receive* from several other neurons simultaneously, thereby increasing the intensity of the message. Neurons learn. In fact, because our genes account for only about 50% of any given trait, experience is key to neural learning and provides for the tremendous *plasticity* of the human brain. Plasticity simply means that the brain is modifiable with daily experience (LeDoux, 2002). The brain thrives on novelty, and familiar or repetitive signals are dampened so that we need not attend consciously to them every time they occur. This simple form of learning allows the neuron to "ignore" the familiar stimulus, thus freeing higher brain centers to work on more important things. Remember the penny in your hand discussed in Chapter 3? The feel of your clothing, the pressure on your feet against the ground, or the constant hum of the refrigerator are all discounted to place a check on the awareness of neural chatter. All of this background stimulation is simply the *context* of life. Should the familiar become novel, as when the refrigerator suddenly clunks instead of hums, then the neurons become sensitized to pass the new, potentially important information along for processing and interpretation. For many children with sensory processing disorder (SPD), the inability to habituate effectively to familiar sensation and a tendency toward a conscious response to the contextual information of the environment may create a learning barrier (Davies & Gavin, 2007; Mangeot et al., 2001).

With so many neural connections in the CNS, how does the brain prevent electrical messages from randomly zipping back and forth along the connected nerve cells? Simple. Nerve cells are not connected, and they only allow for one-way conduction (Kandel & Siegelbaum, 2000). The brain does this by breaking the connection between neurons by creating a little gap called a *synapse*. Now the CNS has a problem to solve. How does a message traverse the gap? It does so through a release of chemicals called *neurotransmitters* that drift the information across the synaptic space toward the next nerve cell. Now the message has become *electrical-chemical* and will become electrical-chemical-electrical if the next neuron fires as a result of stimulation by the neurotransmitters (LeDoux, 2002). All of this happens in fractions of seconds. Further organization is achieved by a balance between these chemicals, some of which excite the next cell, and some of which inhibit the next cell from firing. Fine tuning is not yet complete. *Neuromodulators*, additional chemicals produced in the brainstem, bathe the brain with supplementary influence, calming or alerting the system globally. Neurotransmitters include serotonin, dopamine, epinephrine, and norepinephrine. *Hormones* can also be added to the mix for even more modification as necessary.

Returning to the description of the classroom, the chatter has become overwhelming, but the students are still expected to converse with one another within a constructivist learning activity. Their progress needs monitoring, but discrete conversations cannot be discerned. When all of the sound has blended into a cacophony of auditory sensation, children can be asked to use "indoor voices." That would be one effective strategy. Another would be for the teacher to circulate the classroom and come closer to each group to make specific conversations more distinguishable. As the teacher moves around, each separate discussion is differentiated, and the teamwork of students is praised.

The CNS uses a similar strategy. The more a group of neurons fires together, the more the neurons become linked into *circuits*, much like the groups of students in the classroom. When neural circuits work together, they become *systems* that perform a specific function, such as hearing or vision (LeDoux, 2002). By connecting neurons into circuits, functional structures in the brain are also connected, and the features of sensation, movement, and cognition interact for an adaptive behavioral response. When actively engaged in the physical or social environment, no event is just sensory, motor, cognitive, or emotional. Integration is a key feature of learning, behaving, and remembering. Indeed, the brain is organization upon organization.

Sometimes, however, these intricate strategies do not seem to operate with efficiency, and circuits become disordered. The inefficiency of an important circuit connecting certain parts of the brain may be implicated in a number of neurobehavioral disorders of childhood, including attention-deficit/hyperactivity disorder (ADHD), pervasive developmental disorder (PDD), Asperger syndrome, and autism (Melillo & Leisman, 2004). That these disabilities often share common symptoms, such as attention-deficit, poor motor coordination, and sensory processing difficulty, may offer testimony to the highly integrated nature of brain function and, therefore, to the wide ranging effect of various degrees and locations of dysfunction in brain structures and neural circuits.

MOVEMENT, LEARNING, AND THE FAR AND NEAR SENSES

There is no arguing the connection between learning and the visual and auditory senses, sometimes called the *far senses*. Everyone is familiar with taste and smell, but successful engagement in any occupation, whether movement, social, or academic, is dependent on the effective processing of *all* sensation, including tactile, proprioceptive, and vestibular. This relates to the previous discussion of the cerebellum and its dual engagement in the processing of sensation for movement control, as well as tasks involving mental arithmetic, mental imagery, mental word and word use association, motivation, emotion, and memory.

The execution of goal-directed movement for occupational engagement in the classroom further combines the processing of sensation with the planning and monitoring functions of the prefrontal executive. This is known as *praxis,* or *motor planning,* and it allows for the conceptualization, organization, and sequencing of nonhabitual or novel actions (Reeves & Cermak,

2002). Refined dexterity and haptic perception are diminished without accurate tactile ability to feel objects for adjustment and manipulation.

Spatial learning is mediated in part by the engagement of the body in the environment, and binary concepts, such as hot and cold, left and right, and fast and slow, are grounded in sensation and movement. Skill-based learning is gained implicitly through the movement–learning link and is embedded artfully in educational best practice.

Sensory information is fed to the emotion centers of the brain for evaluation of content for danger and is shipped to the memory centers where perceptions converge to produce multisensory conceptions (LeDoux, 2002). Without the ability to process and integrate the sensory elements of the environment, *red, round,* and *sweet* would never become *apple,* and abstract thought would have no foundation. Without the ability to reconstruct and consolidate the various sensory components of a past event, long-term memories would just be independent fragments of sight or sound or taste.

Occupational therapists (OTs) are fond of using the terms *near senses* or *power senses* in describing the tactile, vestibular, and proprioceptive sensory channels and prioritizing them because they are foundational. Both teachers and OTs are concerned with the processing of domain-specific visual and auditory information for conscious learning and movement control. The near senses, however, underlie movement and the individual's *readiness* for learning and action, and they are substantial factors in the movement–learning link.

Tactile sensation travels from the periphery to the brain along different neural pathways, depending on the particular stimulus (Gertz, 2007). Pain and temperature, for example, are carried separately from awareness of texture, shape, and size. This makes sense because one pathway is protective, and requires a quick and crude response. The other is discriminative and recognizes the differences among type, quality, and location of touch and can be a partner in the learning of language and math concepts through haptic activities. The sensory processing area of the cortex creates a body map based on touch and informs the young child of the physical boundaries of self and the difference between *me* and *you* or *me* and *it.* Touch links self emotionally with others, directs fine motor activity, and provides a soothing source of regulation in times of distress.

Vestibular and proprioceptive messages contribute to the active movement of the body through space, the maintenance of posture and balance, the steadiness of gait, muscle tone, and some eye movement. By helping to keep the child upright and alert, they may become one regulator of the attentional readiness of students. In addition to touch, these sensory channels organize the body to connect with environment and task; powerfully deliver a calming, self-regulatory influence; and are recruited heavily in the treatment of SPD. Information through the near or power senses is encoun-

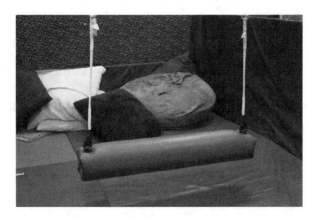

tered in virtually every educational act, and much of it is silently or subconsciously processed for mastery in the classroom. Sensation is food for the movement–learning link.

SENSORY PROCESSING
AND THE ADAPTIVE RESPONSE

Sensory processing is never just sensory. If the goal is to engage successfully in purposeful and meaningful occupation, then an *adaptive response* will be necessary. Depending on the circuit traveled and the brain centers activated, the sensory information is analyzed, compared, and interpreted and then sent to be thought about and acted on. Raising a hand to answer questions in class is different than chasing a soccer ball, and it is definitely different from the response required when smoke is detected in a room. Thus, a behavioral response is adaptive when it is an appropriate match to the demands of the environment or task and enables occupational performance (Kimball, 1999). Sensory self-regulation is different than the term as it used by teachers. Teachers often refer to self-regulation as planning, organizing, self-monitoring, help seeking, and goal setting as managed by the executive functions of the prefrontal cortex. Sensory self-regulation is aligned more closely to the primary sensory foundations of achieving and maintaining baseline arousal and producing the adaptive response. Although the two are interrelated and interdependent, the underlying assumptions and interventional strategies are unique.

A response can serve a purpose and yet not be adaptive. When a young child refuses to touch paint or playdough, his or her response may serve a need to avoid an objectionable tactile sensation, but it may not be adaptive for engagement in the classroom art project. When a lethargic child suddenly bursts into disruptive activity, such a response may serve a need to increase baseline arousal, but it certainly is not adaptive when the teacher is quietly reading a book to the group. Determination of the adaptiveness of response to sensation and detective work regarding the barriers and contributors to successful occupational performance within various contexts is at the heart of sensory processing theory, assessment, and intervention.

The adaptiveness of response can be placed on a continuum from low to high and passive to active (Reeves, 2001). The active response does not refer to the movement of the body, but rather to children's level of engagement in a goal-directed, purposeful action, whether they are reading silently or launching themselves down a slide. On the passive end, children may, for example, be held and rocked for calming. When ready, they will show a more active adaptive response by reengaging and participating happily and independently in the opportunities of a sensory rich environment. Support for children who show low level adaptive response will draw them carefully and gradually toward successful play and performance in all tasks and environments.

THEORY, TERMINOLOGY, AND CONFIRMATION OF SENSORY PROCESSING DISORDER

Sensory integration is the original theory and the legacy of Dr. A. Jean Ayres (1923–1988). Dr. Ayres was an OT and educational psychologist with additional training in neuroscience who proposed a relationship between internal neural processes and the behavioral responses of children with learning challenges and disabilities. Because sensory integration in the brain could not be seen directly, Ayres drew inferences about dysfunctional motor, learning, and social-emotional behavioral patterns and theorized that the effective interpretation and synthesis of sensation enabled the child to engage effectively in a given environment (Ayres, 1972). Much like the sensory processing of auditory or visual information, which has implications for learning, Ayres presumed that the processing of the sensory foundations of movement would have similar implications. Certain kinds of observed behavioral dysfunction in children with learning disabilities, such as poorly planned and executed motor action, were therefore assumed to reflect a level of internal neural disorganization in the brain's use of sensory messages.

Because movement both generates and encounters sensation, it is considered to be one of the most powerful organizers of adaptive behavior and continues to be a central feature of sensory integration intervention. Ayres theorized about the movement–learning link long before its confirmation by neuroscience technologies in the decade of the brain, and her assumptions based on observation are now receiving scrutiny and validation through contemporary study based on new scientific methodologies (Davies & Gavin, 2007; Miller, Coll, & Schoen, 2007). Indeed, children with SPD have been found to have difficulty filtering or suppressing repeated sensory signals and respond to sensation more variably than children without SPD. In recent research, children with SPD were distinguished from typically developing children with 86% accuracy using measures of electrical brain activity (Davies & Gavin, 2007). Furthermore, continued rigorous research on discrete intervention outcomes has found that occupational therapy services for children with SPD resulted in significant gains in several outcome measures when compared with those receiving alternative or no services (Miller, Coll, et al., 2007).

Sensory processing is the term used to refer to the entire neurobehavioral loop, which includes the nervous system's use of sensory input and the resulting behavioral response. SPD is suspected when the response to sensory events is not adaptive and thus significantly interferes with the individual's ability to successfully engage in daily life occupations, whether dressing, playing, working, or completing the educational tasks of school (Miller, Anzalone, Lane, Cermak, & Osten, 2007). The prevalence of SPD is estimated as at least 5.3% and possibly as high as 13.7% among children of kindergarten age in the general population (Ahn, Miller, Milberger, & McIntosh, 2004). SPD frequently coexists with other childhood neurobehavioral disorders, including autism, PDD, Asperger syndrome, and ADHD.

Everyone has sensory preferences. Many people reject certain foods based on taste or texture. Some like to work with the radio on, others turn it off. Intense movement makes me dizzy, and you will not find me on amusement park rides. My personal responses to sensation have contributed to the person I am—a little on the sedentary side, preferring to work in a quiet room, fond of tomatoes but definitely not beets. These are minor challenges, however, and do not prevent me from engaging in daily tasks or meeting the demands of the environment. The child who is highly sensitive to sound cannot adapt to the demands of a school band concert. The child who is very sensitive to touch may fall apart during dressing or grooming routines. The child with poor postural stability may avoid active sports, even though participation is desperately desired. SPD is not a matter of strong sensory preferences. It is debilitating for the child and challenging for the caregiver and teacher. It requires serious consideration, along with careful management of the child's activities and environment. *Sensory rich* should be *sensory satisfying* for all children.

Generally, well-conceived plans of appropriate activity are best offered both at school *and* at home, as children with SPD require a comprehensive approach. Research suggests that sensory processing patterns may be fairly stable across the lifespan and tend to interact with temperament and personality (Dunn, 2001). They are at the core of who we are as unique individuals. Insight gained from an understanding of sensory patterns and the strategies that enable effective occupational performance is invaluable to individuals, teachers, and families.

ASSESSMENT OF SUSPECTED
SENSORY PROCESSING DISORDER

When a child is unable to engage successfully in the occupations of the school routines, and adaptive response is elusive, the evaluation team may initiate a series of multidisciplinary assessments. The OT will want to schedule observations to begin a dynamic assessment of the child's daily performance in the context of various school environments. It is also likely that the OT will want to interview the teacher and request that a profile of the child's typical responses to representative sensory encounters be completed. Any behavioral documentation will be valuable to the therapist because it may provide clues to the child's responsiveness to environment and task, as well as social aptitude. If the child has an IEP, the OT will guide the intervention strategies with teacher feedback. If the child is not eligible for special education services, the evaluation summary may include recommendations for classroom modifications and natural accommodations to help the child to participate more successfully. If the child is transferring from another school district or transitioning from preschool to kindergarten, any known effective strategies should be in place for arrival on day one.

PATTERNS OF SENSORY PROCESSING DISORDER

Everyone experiences variations in arousal levels during the day. We may become fidgety during a long meeting or drowsy after lunch. A sudden unexpected sound may startle us, temporarily heightening our alertness and causing us to jump. Our heart rate increases, and we may breathe a little harder. After a few minutes, we are able to return to the *midrange* level of arousal and can continue effectively with our current task. These variations are perfectly suited to the sensory conditions within our bodies and the environment and, therefore, contribute to the adaptive response. Each of us also has a repertoire of sensory strategies that serve to maintain the match between attentional and emotional responses and the task demands. When we are drowsy during the day, our strategies may include stretching, having a cold drink, opening a window, or finding a novel activity. When we need to stay alert during a meeting, we may jiggle our foot or doodle or chew gum. If we need to calm ourselves, curling up on the sofa, wrapping in a blanket, or having a warm cup of tea may do the trick.

Most of us have a natural awareness of three core principles for the effective application of sensory strategies—*intensity, frequency,* and *duration* (Williams & Shellenburger, 1996). When we are in significant need of calming or organizing, a light pat on the back simply won't do, but a deep and enduring hug will. A long and intense physical workout will relieve the tensions of the day, and frequent forms of exercise will maintain tranquility over time. The proactive timing of sensory strategies will make all the difference in sustaining occupational performance or reestablishing adaptive response for children who show escalating behavior. For the child with SPD, these three principles must be managed and applied thoughtfully with carefully designed strategies to support occupational performance in school.

The regulation of adaptive behavior can involve strategies other than sensory, and all can be imposed by either ourselves (self-regulation) or others along the adaptive response continuum. *Cognitive strategies* involve higher level thinking and might include learned social constraints, such as "I must not hit my friends" or "I use a quiet voice in the classroom." *Behavioral strategies* generally involve a reward or consequence, whether immediate, delayed, or perceived, and might be applied in the form of if-then instructions (e.g., "If I do my work, then I will get a break."). When cognitive and behavioral strategies fail, as when the child is in distress and is not receptive to reasoning, sensory strategies may constitute the most successful intervention and are particularly effective as a preventive measure for children with SPD. When teachers, behavior specialists, and OTs are available as interventionists on the same education team, careful collaboration will be necessary to determine the most effective application of all strategies. Given the appropriate supports and accommodations, children with SPD should show gradual improvement in adaptive response and can be weaned away from many strategies over time.

Children who are alert, relaxed, and focused in the classroom are in a state of learning readiness. They are actively engaged, even if the activity is silent reading or listening. They, too, find sensory strategies to maintain both arousal and motor preparedness for task, although adults may initially help them to choose those that are most appropriate or direct the elements of intensity, frequency and duration. Teachers become attuned to the energy levels of the group and know when to modify an activity to recapture students' attention. For adults and children with typical sensory processing, adaptive responses are the rule and minor variations of arousal and readiness are managed seamlessly throughout the day. This is a difficult challenge for some children, however, and at some point in every career it is likely that a teacher will be responsible for the education of a child whose sensory processing patterns create barriers to learning. Each of the three response patterns in relation to environment, routine, task, and social encounters are discussed next with the understanding that they vary in severity and can be present in various combinations in a single child.

Sensory Modulation Disorder

Children with sensory modulation disorder (SMD) are at a distinct disadvantage in the complex environment of the classroom, and their behavior seems rarely to be well matched to the task demands. They may manifest responses that indicate *sensory overresponsivity*, *sensory underresponsivity*, or *sensory-seeking behavior*, each of which is a subtype of SMD (Miller, Coll, et al., 2007). It is important to remember that children with SMD may respond well to cognitive and/or linguistic strategies (e.g., social stories) or behavioral interventions that include if-then reasoning or reward and consequence, but only when arousal makes them receptive and their learning readiness is ensured.

The Overresponsive Child

Classrooms are inherently stimulating places, and the control of every sensory component is not possible. However, it is important to know that the effects of the sensory stimulants from the environment are cumulative, and we are not necessarily aware of their influence. Children with SMD cannot easily reset their arousal level, and any response to a sensory event can leave them vulnerable out of the developmentally appropriate midrange. The child with sensory *overresponsivity* may respond intensely to a sensation that seems benign to others. The touch of glue, the scratchiness of embroidery on a T-shirt, the hum of the fluorescent lighting, and the movement of peers around them can all elicit an emotional outburst that requires urgent management. The sensory culprit may be obvious, as with the glue, and the child's response immediate. Yet, arousal can also build gradually and without the ability to reset to midrange, any common occurrence can elicit an explosive behavior that seems to come out of the blue. Overresponsive children can be challenged by a single sensory modality (e.g., touch or sound) or to multiple modalities, and they are unlikely to be able to verbalize their resulting feelings or explain the emotions that overwhelm them.

Over time, teachers and caregivers will become alert to signs of behavioral escalation and can then intervene quickly to relieve the anxious child. Such signs might include an increase in body movement (for children with autism, this may come in the form of hand flapping or pacing); fretful facial expression; or repetitive vocalizations that may increase in volume. When engaging overresponsive children, approach from the side or front so that they can anticipate the interaction.

Vigilance is a normal and functional condition of the nervous system and refers to the preparedness or readiness of the system to receive sensory input for use. Children with overresponsive patterns can be *hypervigilant*, which has survival value and is adaptive in extreme or threatening circumstances. This is the point—overresponsive children may frequently feel threatened and are ever expectant of a sensory assault. Yet, hypervigilance comes at a cost. In a complex environment, such as the classroom, there are many opportunities for sensory encounters, and oversensitive children may appear to be distracted or off task. Actually, they are in significant self-protection mode, may miss instructional cues as a result, and may be unreceptive or unable to apply cognitive or behavioral regulations. The distracted state can also be a sign that arousal is heightened, placing the child precariously close to a magnified response to the next sensory event.

Children with sensory overresponsivity may show two different behavioral patterns (Miller, Coll, et al., 2007). In the first pattern, they may at times show physical refusal or physical or verbal aggression, crying, anxiety, and impulsivity. This is not behavior that responds to reason or other traditional strategies, and trying to "talk them down" may not be successful. It is not willful behavior; rather, it can be a fight-or-flight response, and no matter how illogical it may seem, it must be understood as physiological, subconscious, and quite reasonable in its own way.

A second pattern (more likely on a continuum of behavioral responses) may include fearfulness and withdrawal. Overresponsive children are often described as controlling and rigid, and they may demand sameness of food, clothing, toys, or routines. This makes eminent sense as an avoidance pattern and protects the child against potentially intolerable sensory encounters. Gradual introduction to novel or sensory-loaded experiences helps this child to tolerate a wider variety of activities. For example, watching the action of the group may be followed by alternative participation, such as taking notes or reading instructions, and may lead to even greater engagement on the child's own terms.

School Environment and the Overresponsive Child

Teachers may want to take a renewed look at the environment of the classroom through the eyes of a child with sensory overresponsiveness and with the understanding that the sensory environment also influences the learning and productivity of the typically developing child. The color of the walls, the number of things *on* the walls and hanging from the ceiling, the acoustics of the room, and the lighting all represent bits of sensory information that must be processed, much of it simultaneously. Reds and oranges are alerting to most people and may push the overresponsive child out of midrange over time. Blues and greens are calming.

The sheer number of visual images in a classroom can create a summative sensory effect on arousal. It is wise to have at least one wall remain fairly clear and neutral, particularly the one behind the dry erase board or behind the teacher's favored location when addressing the class. In this way, children's visual attention is not diverted or distributed when instruction is given. Book shelves or storage cubbies can be covered with fabric curtains in a calming color, thus not only eliminating a vast number of visual stimulants, but also replacing them with a single, neutralizing surface. If cubbies cannot be covered, the organization of materials into containers of the same size, shape, and color can lend visual uniformity to the classroom. Lighting, generally fluorescent, can be annoying to some and can be supplemented with lamplight, particularly with "daylight" bulbs or full-spectrum lighting. If natural light is available in the classroom, then I often recommend turning the overhead lights off on a sunny day. With an overresponsive child in the classroom, avoid blinking the lights as an attention bridge.

The auditory environment can be difficult to control. School bells can be loud and piercing, although many schools have modified their tone. Teachers may clap or ring a chime to orient the children to instruction or task. Any auditory strategies may require some preventive modification because an immediate response to a single sound may not be forthcoming from the overresponsive child. For children who are instantly sensitive to sound (they may frequently put hands over ears), peers can be instructed in the art of "silent clapping" with their finger tips. Noise-reduction headphones may help the sound-sensitive child to concentrate, although the touch-sensitive child may not want to wear them! Nature sound audio CDs or beat-per-second musical backgrounds may be worth a try. Classical music and Native American rhythm CDs are commercially available for just this purpose. It is important to also remember that adults are part of the environment and our reassuring voices are calming and organizing.

A respite corner will provide the overresponsive child with occasional relief from the activity of the classroom (see Figure 5.1). A large beanbag chair or even a pile of large pillows may work well. A small child's tent may help reduce the light and visual distraction. Many schools have designated sensory rooms designed by the OT that, in addition to therapy sessions, can be reserved for supervised respite at regular intervals during the day.

Make sure to consider all environments of the school, as each presents a unique sensory challenge. Music rooms can be particularly difficult and large open cafeterias can reverberate sound and contain many more children

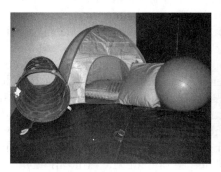 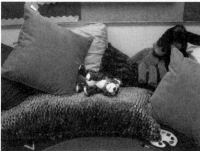

Figure 5.1. Respite corners in a classroom.

than the sensory sensitive child can tolerate. Playgrounds, hallways, and staircases can be a jumble of movement and sound. Even the school bus is an environment of its own, and its sensory elements can prepare the child for an uneventful day or set the stage for disaster from the moment of arrival. With careful planning and a compassionate eye on the environment and its sensory components, the overresponsive child can enjoy a safe and supportive school experience.

Social and Academic Engagement and the Overresponsive Child

Overresponsivity to touch can inadvertently "exile" a child from many academic and social activities in the classroom. Much of the time, trial-and-error experimentation may be required in providing materials that will be tolerated and will enable the child to remain part of the group. At other times, the supportive role as reader or director will provide an opportunity for effective engagement. It is important *not* to settle for allowing the overresponsive child to "sit out" most activities, but to collaborate on nonthreatening ways to increase participation and improve occupational performance.

Children who are either overresponsive to touch or to movement may poorly tolerate close proximity with peers and may be hypervigilant during transitions or beginning and end of day routines. They may work more effectively when provided extra workspace at the end of a table or in a study carrel of their own. The movement sensitive child should be monitored closely during recess and PE to ensure gradual or alternative engagement. The child who is sensitive to touch may be more comfortable sitting on the periphery of the group at circle times or may prefer to sit in a chair or other prescribed seating (e.g., a dynamic cushion, carpet square, rocking chair, inflatable stool).

Try to anticipate the more chaotic times of the school day, as they can be particularly traumatic for the overresponsive child. Some preplanning can make all the difference in making the day go smoothly. It often works well to allow the 5-minute early arrival or dismissal time for overresponsive children who can remove or don coat and backpack before peers surround them. Because every day can be a little different (e.g., music on Mondays, computer lab on Wednesdays), making the routine as predictable as possible is important for hypervigilant children. General picture or word schedules help them to anticipate a change in activity and prepare them for transitions. For the child who does not "read" a picture or word schedule, provide a consistent object cue, such as a small instrument that is carried to music class or a book that is toted to the library. Request advanced notice of fire drills and use matter-of-fact tone of voice to prepare the child in advance. Place a special picture on the daily schedule for such an atypical event. The unexpected absence of a teacher or favored paraeducator can have an impact on the entire day. Try to prepare children when they step off the bus, perhaps even keeping a picture of a regular substitute teacher so that it can be carried from bus to classroom. The overresponsive child may need several days to prepare for anticipated changes in routine, such as field trips, concerts, parties, or special assemblies, and may require additional sensory supports or modified expectations during these occasional and novel activities.

Overresponsive children may have difficulty standing or walking in a line. Placing them at the beginning or end will provide some extra space and protect from excessive or unanticipated sensation. Make them the special door holder, as this will allow them to participate, but will prevent incidental touch or movement encounters. Although full participation is the goal, gradual introduction to highly sensory-rich classes such as music or PE may be necessary. Watching or listening from outside the room may have to be a good starting point. Sound filtering headphones or teacher's helper roles are also good beginning strategies.

Modified task demands will likely be necessary. The overresponsive child may not be able to tolerate the feel of paper maché, but may happily tear the paper strips and hand them to a friend. Parents of overresponsive children will be the first to understand the need to adapt, so try not to be overly concerned when an alternative product goes home. Many other strategies will be forthcoming for the child who has an IEP because the OT will know what to try.

The unpredictable movement, touch, and voice elevation of young children can frequently take sensory overresponsive children by surprise; however, isolation from peers is an untenable and often inadvertent alternative. Supporting the child with adaptive seating, modified role expectations, and other strategies from a *sensory diet* (discussed later in this chapter) will increase the likelihood that an overresponsive child will remain with the group for longer periods of time. For example, whereas they may not be able to tolerate hand holding during a circle game, they may be willing to "link" to the group with a short "lifeline" (holding onto one side of a small rigid hoop while a peer holds the other side), and this may be socially preferable to the intervening adult by preserving the peer-to-peer interaction. In addition, arranging quieter turn-taking games on the playground may entice participation.

Children whose behavioral responses are rigid may have a difficult time playing in large groups in which the rules are invented or changed frequently. When the game moves too quickly or when the rules are not their own, they can quickly become demanding of their peers and, thus, damage social relationships. Simply encouraging engagement in an activity that is not so bound by social rules (e.g., climbing or rolling a ball) may be a more tolerable alternative.

In the community, overresponsive children may best be guided toward individualized sports and activities with family or small groups of friends, such as climbing, hiking, swimming, track and field, dance, or bike riding, which will provide them with resistive and organizing movement sensation and will protect them from the unpredictable and dissonant activity of a large group. Rotary movement of the head in space is one of the most stimulating forms of vestibular sensation. Therefore, any sport that requires constant visual searching and monitoring (e.g., soccer, basketball) may be highly disorganizing and intolerable, especially for the overresponsive or hypervigilant child.

When assigning seating, overresponsive children may best be paired with a child whose temperament is on the gentle side and whose behavior is predictable. Providing a location in the front of the room will eliminate extraneous visual stimulation. A seat in the back of the room, however, might allow standing and stretching when needed. It can be a matter of trial and error within a repertoire of appropriate strategies.

To preserve and foster the confidence and self-esteem of overresponsive children, adults must be alert for daily opportunities to let them shine. These are children who often become more adept at thinking through a problem, rather than engaging in physical experimentation. While standing back from the activities of the group, they may be quite capable as class presenters. A natural tendency to observe can give them the opportunity to understand the whole picture, and they may be wonderful resources for explanations and the retelling of events. Overresponsive children may eventually become delegators and can develop excellent managerial skills.

☀ Jeremy ☀

Jeremy is a perfect example of the density and diversity of designed supports and the gradual benefit to adaptive response. His ability to meet behavioral expectations was elusive from the moment he stood in the morning arrival line outside the classroom door, and he was in trouble almost daily for hitting and poking his peers. This behavior continued as he made his way to the cubbies, and unpacking his belongings was accompanied by further aggressive verbal and physical outbursts. Sensitive to touch, sound, and movement, Jeremy could not manage the close proximity of other children at his worktable or on the carpet at circle time. Simply, the school day was very unpleasant for Jeremy, his classmates, and a patient and long-suffering kindergarten teacher. The education team immediately began to put strategies into place. Arrangements were made to transport Jeremy to and from school in a smaller and quieter school bus, and he was allowed early entrance and dismissal to take care of his belong-

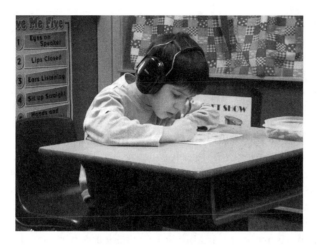

ings. These two accommodations alone changed the tenor of the morning and effectively eliminated significant grounds for hypervigilance. He was additionally provided with a delineated space on the carpet and given fidget toys, a weighted lap pad, a weighted wrap on his chair, and a rocking chair. His desk was moved slightly away from his peers, and he proudly claimed his own "office" space.

Noise-reduction earphones were accessible near his table. Given pictures of children in various arousal states, Jeremy learned to identify his own state when asked. Low demand tasks were assigned to him, and alternative educational and social engagement strategies were designed. With arousal closer to midrange, he responded to a token system, participated in the general classroom behavior plan, began to internalize and inconsistently manifest learned cognitive strategies, and could often be heard repeating the classroom rules. As Jeremy's responses became increasingly matched to the demands of environment and task, a much happier little boy emerged.

The Underresponsive Child

Many general principles were addressed in the previous section regarding the overresponsive child. The following sections address further specific considerations for children who are underresponsive and sensory seeking.

The arousal level of *underresponsive* children may appear to be stuck under the midrange, and their posture and affect may reflect apparent apathy or lethargy. They can be described as self-absorbed when, in fact, their unique sensory-and-response system precludes an outward orientation. The underresponsive child may not be as susceptible as the overresponsive child to emotional outbursts and may not require behavior crisis management in the classroom. Yet more subtle performance concerns are noted and reported by the teacher, who frequently finds a need to reexplain missed oral instruction, to call attention to overlooked written cues, or to direct several attention prompts to a child who appears not to hear.

As with all children with SPD, the underresponsive child is generally not willfully uncooperative. Rather, the sensory-rich encounters of the classroom that are stimulating and alerting to most children are not registered or used effectively to achieve and sustain learning readiness for successful adaptive response and occupational performance. In contrast to the overresponsive child, the arousal of an underresponsive child can decline gradually during long phases of concentrated academics, and efficient and independent initiation of work may prove to be inconsistent or impossible. Teachers may report the child's apparent forgetfulness, solitary and sedentary play tendencies, lack of motivation, or inability to get ideas on paper. Routine tasks, such as putting materials away or pushing in a chair, may require daily reminders well beyond the learning time frame required by most of the other children.

Teachers may find that they become inadvertently bound to a prompt-dependent relationship with the underresponsive child, who shows limited anticipatory preparedness and limited natural vigilance. In fact, a need for inordinate cueing to transition this child efficiently will often motivate an appeal to the special services evaluation team.

Underresponsive children, however, can present with an alternative self-management tendency that can challenge performance and create a learning barrier. They may swing inconsistently toward bursts of activity in an effort to reset their low arousal, and they may require sensory strategies similar to those of the sensory-seeking child. Creative embedding of frequent and intense sensory options that heighten alerting sensation can help to balance the underresponsive child's ability to engage productively in the educational environment.

School Environment and
the Underresponsive Child

For the underresponsive child to register a behavioral response to sensation, it will need to be more intense, more frequent, or of longer duration. However, rather than ramping up the entire classroom environment with bright colors and lively sound, a more effective approach is to concentrate alerting sensation by calling discrete attention to a specific task or activity. For example, placing a bright placemat on the table will rivet attention to a spelling task. Providing worksheets with unusual, bold, italicized, underlined, color-highlighted, or larger fonts will call attention to salient instructional information. A tactile surface under a coloring paper (e.g., fine needlepoint grid) may increase the child's interest and extend participation. Providing dynamic seating options, such as cushions that encourage dynamic engagement of the body core in multiple movement planes, will help to alert the postural system and increase the baseline level of arousal. Attention bridges that incorporate sound (e.g., clapping patterns, chimes) may work well for underresponsive children. Even in stimulating environments, however, they may not engage and regularly embedded alerting supports will be necessary throughout the day.

Social and Academic
Engagement and the Underresponsive Child

Sensory underresponsive children can also be self-isolating. They may not orient to their name; respond to *distant cues* (e.g., verbal cues delivered to the group from across the room); or respond to ambient cues that signal a transition. For example, they may continue to play or work quietly while the other children are lining up at the door, or they may lag behind their peers during a song with accompanying gestures. Instructional cues, which often must be repeated might better be delivered in close proximity from the front and preceded by a gentle but firm alerting touch to the arm or shoulder. Visual timers placed nearby may offer an additional cue to the timing of transitions. Manipulatives and move-and-learn activities are particularly supportive of learning. Extended periods of sedentary work, such as listening to a story or watching a DVD, can further decelerate underresponsive children. Allowing them to read along with a copy of the teacher's book can keep them engaged and listening during quiet times. Alerting options from a sensory diet will support participation and may range from fidget toys to movement breaks. Recess and PE will feed arousal, but successful involvement may still require careful planning. Peers may lose interest when attempting to engage the underresponsive child, whose social isolation is at great risk. Undoubtedly there are patient, persistent, and demonstrative peers who would be the perfect play or work partners and whose leadership qualities naturally incline them to help and guide.

Although appearing somewhat aloof, underresponsive children may enjoy delving deeply into an academic subject and can be recruited as class experts on their favorite line of study. They may be the perfect choice for a novel and independent project that builds confidence in their unique abilities, especially if they can later present their findings to the class. A balance between social engagement and self-direction is a reasonable goal for underresponsive children, and they will gradually be recognized and admired by their peers.

The Sensory-Seeking Child

All young children can be overly active and difficult to calm at times. Sensory-seeking children take engagement to the extreme, however, and always seem to crave intensity, whether in food flavors, sound (often self-produced), movement, or touch. They may try very hard to show midrange behavior during quiet times in school, but their underlying sensory patterns may reflect general underresponsiveness, and they may cope by bursting unexpectedly into a frenzy of activity to adjust their arousal. Fine tuning, such as stretching or temporary fidgeting, may not be enough, and dramatic shifts in behavior are possible. They will miss instruction when actively searching for sensory encounters, which may drive them to leave their seats, engage peers, and fiddle with materials on their way to the teacher. "Get out your pencil" will send them on extended explorations inside their desks. Their bodies just cannot be still. ADHD may be the first diagnostic suspect and can actually co-occur with SPD. If sufficient stimulation is not forthcoming from environment or task, sensory-seeking children are likely to manufacture it themselves. "Listening" postures are only briefly held, and sensory seekers may stand, sprawl over the desk, sit awkwardly over their feet, or perch precariously on the edge of the chair in an unconscious effort to intensify sensory signals through the body. Oral strategies are readily accessible, and pencils or shirtsleeves can be constantly in the mouth. Self-stimulatory vocalizations such as humming, or impulsive behaviors such as reaching for displayed materials, may disrupt the class and result in disciplinary action by the teacher. Expect pens to be tapped on the table, papers to be shuffled, and feet to wiggle. The trend toward longer quiet and sedentary periods in the classroom is not a good match for the young sensory-seeking child who has both a developmental and a sensory-based need for active engagement. Recess is a necessity for this child. Remember that the often disorganized search for sensation serves a *purpose*, although sensory-seeking children may not articulate their sensory needs and they cannot answer the "why" question. Multidisciplinary evaluations will help to sort out the executive attention-deficit from sensory-based seeking behavior.

Environment and the Sensory-Seeking Child

The environment of sensory-seeking children must be highly preemptive, providing opportunities for engagement in sensory rich experience that will satisfy their need for stimulation and prevent frequent bursts into seeking behavior that is disruptive. They must be heavily supported during quiet work times with strategies such as dynamic seating, fidget toys, weighted vests or lap pads, and intensely flavored or textured snacks.

The principles of intensity, frequency, and duration of sensory engagement require regular consideration, particularly in fine tuning the sensory-

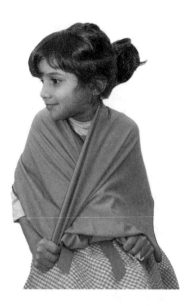

seeking child's sensory diet. For example, fidget toys may satisfy a need for duration, but not for intensity. Visits to the sensory room may satisfy the need for intensity, which is at a premium there, but may not address frequency. Visits can be strategically placed into the daily schedule, however. Resistive fidget toys, such as those that can be squeezed, bent, or stretched, will heighten the sensation and may more readily satisfy the child's cravings.

Be cognizant of the sensory properties of classroom materials and their effect on the behavior of the sensory-seeking child. Lightweight materials, such as rice in the texture table, can either provide needed tactile sensation or may conversely fail to constrain engagement and appropriate play. On the other hand, materials and tasks that offer weight and resistance, including dragging the ball bin, pushing the book cart, or stacking chairs on tables, will reduce the need for seeking behavior. Embed more structured movement and transitions in learning activities. Be creative and preemptive in anticipating the sensory seeker's limit within a quiet activity or bring in a rocking chair to extend engagement and sustain attention. Be generous in allowing changes of position, and offer a variety of alternatives by designing a respite corner and providing space to stretch out on the floor.

Social and Academic
Engagement and the Sensory-Seeking Child

Active learning tasks can be well suited to the sensory seekers, although a caution is offered. Whereas they crave sensation, they may not be able to organize their behavior as the activity level escalates. It is not a simple matter of activity, but the *right* activity that will feed a seeking system and enable organized and successful participation. These children may initially need special assignments or opportunities during inherently dynamic recess or PE, particularly for pursuits incorporating heavy work to muscles and joints. For example, encouragement to climb on the playground big toys rather than join a fast-paced and unpredictable game of tag may place needed parameters around activity and movement and ensure an adaptive transition back into the classroom.

Attempts to establish friendships can bring frustration and disappointment to both sensory-seeking children and their peers. During deskwork, they may pester their neighbor. During circle time, they may be constantly touching others. While walking in a line, they may find a great source of proprioception and deep pressure touch by bumping and crashing into friends who may quickly lose their patience. If inadvertently rewarded for silly behavior, the sensory seeker may learn to thrive on the feedback that is elusive in more serious social encounters. Be alert to opportunities; for example, drama class may be a perfect match because of its balance of movement, activity, and structure. Although group games and sports seem to offer good potential for sensation, *individual* sports provide resistive and organized movement and may be better suited to a sensory-seeking child, just as they are also well suited to the overresponsive child. Without regular and appropriate outlets for his or her need to explore and experience, the sensory seeker may resort to excessive and unsafe risk taking and should, therefore, be carefully guided to appropriate movement outlets that might be developed throughout the lifespan.

When the sensory system is satiated and behavioral responses organized and adaptive, sensory-seeking children can be eager participants in novel activities and may be the perfect choice for demonstrating and modeling new instruction. An assignment as teacher's helper can offer movement opportunity and will increase confidence in the child's ability to engage successfully in the educational environment.

Sensory-Based Motor Disorder

Sensory-based motor disorder (SBMD), the second pattern of SPD, implicates an inefficiency of the near senses of tactile, proprioception, and vestibular processing, all of which are integrated for smooth, coordinated, and adjusted motor responses (Miller, Anzalone, et al., 2007). Children with SBMD may have a *postural disorder* characterized by poor muscle tone, stability, balance, and endurance, and they are likely to have a difficult time with postural readiness at their desks. They may alternatively have *dyspraxia*, a deficit in praxis, which combines the functions of intentional skilled movement execution with the cognitive conception, planning, and sequencing of unrehearsed actions. Although children with postural disorder may avoid active games and sports, their challenge is with motor execution rather than with planning. Children with dyspraxia may also be unable to initiate a novel task because they cannot seem to envision the function, sequence, or operation of the objects involved. They do not know the how of an action and can easily become frustrated when things just don't work for them. They do not seem to be flexible in their approach, and they may have a limited repertoire of trial-and-error strategies. The ability to generalize motor learning to new situations may not come easily, and the organization of desk, materials, notebooks, and binders can be frustratingly inefficient. In addition to occupational therapy approaches for the amelioration of sensory dysfunction, children with dyspraxia may also be taught to develop visual, verbal self-cueing, and cognitive problem-solving strategies to help them negotiate an unfamiliar task or routine and systematize the arrangement of their belongings.

Because of the motor implications of these SPDs, children with postural disorder or dyspraxia will need more time to acquire new skills and more practice to develop them. Handwriting, for example, requires complex sequencing and refined movement. Children with SBMD will benefit from a more leisurely pace in the writing process, allowing them more time to develop automaticity with basic patterns before the language elements become more demanding. A balance between independent trial and adult or peer assistance will preserve confidence and self-mastery.

Sensory Discrimination Disorder

Children with sensory discrimination disorder (SDD) have specific difficulty with the ability to perceive similarities and differences in sensory events related to tactile, proprioceptive, and vestibular functioning (Miller, Anzalone, et al., 2007). SDD is thus treated distinctly from visual or auditory processing problems of childhood. Fine or gross motor incoordination is a clue to SDD, although a more discrete dysfunction of haptic perception may indicate a difficulty in the tactile sensory system. Any task that must be tackled without the aid of visual input, such as buttoning a shirt, may prove to be a frustrating challenge. Limited informational sensation from the power or body senses may result in heavy reliance on the visual guidance of movement and may prolong the learning phase of academic tasks, such as handwriting or keyboarding.

Children with SDD may appear slow to acquire procedural skills in relation to peers, and occupational performance may suffer. However, a somewhat awkward motor performance may not preclude an ability to benefit from the educational curriculum in the school environment, and motor difficulty may not reach the threshold for special education evaluation or service. (This is true for any child because as all SPDs differ in severity.) Interventions may remain at the level of core or targeted instruction and may include such accommodations as increased time allowances for motor learning and activities, work reduction, or extra trials. As for all children, a focus on what they do well and guidance toward the best child–task match will preserve self-confidence and maintain motivation to participate and learn.

THE SENSORY DIET

The term *sensory diet* implies several things. First, similar to food and water, it is accessed regularly throughout the day to maintain optimal arousal and function. Second, it is necessary for occupational survival of the child with SPD in the complex, variable, and demanding environments of school and classroom. Third, it is "served" from a menu of *healthy* sensory options prescribed to suit the unique needs of a unique student. Fourth, with experience and training, the child with SPD will learn to choose sensory options independently and wisely for optimal adaptive response in every life context and throughout the lifespan. Finally, the sensory diet is an accommodation, not a contingency program, and should never be provided only as a reward or withheld as a behavioral consequence.

A sensory diet accounts for the personal preferences of the child and can be designed with his or her participation. Sensation through any channel can be alerting and arousing *or* calming and moderating to adaptive behavior, and, thus, no modality need be exempt from the menu. Sound, for example, can be rousing and lively and entice organizing movement from the underresponsive child. It can also be slow and soothing and beguile the overresponsive child to calm and engage. Movement itself, when slow, rhythmic, and linear, can lull us to sleep. When erratic, rotary, or diverse in speed and direction, it will wake us right up and may be just the right offering on the sensory menu of the underresponsive child. Light touch or tickling can be insufferable to the child who is tactile sensitive, although consistent and predictable deep pressure touch may be readily accepted and well-tolerated. The ability to predict sensation and its familiarity to the individual will eliminate much of the anticipatory distraction or anxiety for the child who is hypervigilant.

A crucial and often overlooked component of the sensory diet is *education*. The child with SPD is rarely intuitive about the most effective choices in support of adaptive behavior. No amount of rational verbal coaxing will calm the child who is in fight-or-flight mode and who is frantically searching for any escape or source of consolation. Children who are driven to seek sensation, or who do not respond readily to the natural sensory encounters of the classroom, cannot analyze or appropriately adjust their own behavior patterns. Therefore, facilitation of an early, gradual, and developmentally appropriate understanding of the effects of sensation on behavior, along with confirmation and praise for the wisest sensory strategy choices, will increase the likelihood that every child will, over time, become more independent managers of their own needs and responses.

Education is equally important for peers and compassionately sharing the rationale for special materials and equipment is generally met with great understanding. Teachers sometimes question the fairness of providing attractive materials to one child and not to the others. In my experience, this is generally not an issue for students. Teachers who have experimented with therapy balls for the entire class are often pleasantly surprised at the focused attention and work endurance of all children, which makes this an option. Otherwise, whereas peers can always be offered the opportunity to try out the sensory strategies designed for a classmate, it is likely that such materials will not hold long-lasting allure for the child with typical sensory processing ability.

Designing a Sensory Diet

Because the sensory diet may require frequent adjustment, collaboration between the teaching staff and the OT practitioner is essential. Sensory strategies are dynamic and suited to the child's changing ability to demonstrate a higher level adaptive response. The appendix (see pages 136–142) represents a foundation of shared knowledge focusing on the rationale and expected benefits of sensory modifications and accommodations commonly recommended for the classroom that are frequent components of the sensory diet. These strategies are targeted to the child with SMD. The goal of each strategy is mutual—to enable children with SMD to participate happily and successfully with their peers in the environments and tasks of the educational environment and to become an engaged and lifelong learner.

An effective planning chart, which may enumerate many of these sensory diet options, is developed by the OT in collaboration with the teacher (see Figure 5.2). It is reviewed and modified regularly over the course of the school year and will remind the team to consider the child's routines, transitions, and social opportunities, as well as ways to facilitate academic engagement, which can be calming or alerting, depending on the structure of the activity.

THE PARAEDUCATOR IN THE CLASSROOM

Many children with SPD would simply not make it through the day without a nurturing, patient, and compassionate adult assistant. These indispensable staff members, who are generally part of the special education team, often

☀ ☀ ☀   **Sensory Diet Planning Chart**   ☀ ☀ ☀

Sensory Diet For (name): _____   Date: _____

	Calming	Alerting
Visual		
Auditory		
Tactile		
Movement: Vestibular		
Movement: Proprioception		
Oral		
Routine		
Social opportunity		
Academic engagement		

Teaching the Moving Child: OT Insights that Will Transform Your K–3 Classroom
by Sybil M. Berkey. Copyright © 2009 Paul H. Brookes Publishing Co., Inc. All rights reserved.

Figure 5.2.   Sensory diet planning chart.

come to know their charges better than anyone else and can be a tremendous resource in tracking the child's response to intervention strategies. Consideration of the following guiding principles will facilitate a team approach for the benefit of the child.

- The paraeducator is an integral team member and should be invited to all training sessions about SPD in general or regarding intervention strategies specific to a particular child.

- Although paraeducators suggest many effective and appropriate ideas, they are not responsible for the intervention plan and should never be expected to solve difficult problems or modify the program on their own. Regular and open communication with teachers and specialists is crucial.

- Participation with peers is an essential goal. Modification of environment, task, and routine to benefit the child's optimal occupational engagement are preferable to constant adult assistance. Children can easily become dependent on adult support and may gradually disengage as a result. Based on the team's observations of the child's progress, paraeducators may be able to separate from the child with SPD, even if it simply means sitting farther away during work times.

- Silent gestural cues can sometimes support the child's growing independence more than constant verbal cueing. For example, the child can be provided with a completed project sample and pointing to the parts can remind him of the sequence of steps. A simple picture sequence for "color, cut, and paste" may provide all the cueing needed to complete a project. Reducing the verbal engagement between adult and child will increase the child's opportunity to hear and respond to peer comments and questions and to be alert to teacher instructions and warnings of transitions.

FINAL THOUGHTS

Every student responds uniquely to sensation, and no child is able to maintain optimal learning readiness at every moment of the educational day. Formal assessment of the unique features of children's sensory processing abilities and their adaptive responses across tasks and environments is the responsibility of the OT as a member of the special services evaluation team, and recommended classroom accommodations, modifications, and intervention strategies are implemented in a collaborative model.

Sensory processing, however, is not just about dysfunction and disability. The principles of sensory processing as a foundation for learning can be applied at the level of core instruction to support occupational performance for all children in school. The teacher's awareness of and attention to the link among learning, movement, and the *near* senses (i.e., tactile, vestibular, and proprioception) will engage every child in mind *and* body in support of attention, motivation, participation, and successful educational outcome within a diversely designed and presented curriculum, particularly in the primary grades.

Current research underscores the imperative of collaboration for problem solving and an awareness of various and unique lenses through which we view children professionally. After examining the relationship among SMD, affect, and adaptive behaviors in children diagnosed with Asperger syndrome, Pfeiffer, Kinnealey, Reed, and Herzberg (2005) found significant positive relationships between sensory *hyper*sensitivity and anxiety, as well as *hypo*sensitivity and symptoms of depression. Mangeot and colleagues (2001) identified high correlations between aggressive behavior and tactile sensitivity and sensation-seeking in children with ADHD. Mangeot also found that delinquent behavior and somatic (bodily) complaints were highly correlated with sensation seeking and movement sensitivity, respectively.

The lesson is becoming increasingly clear. A singular line of assumptions, whether behavioral or sensory, may overlook underlying causal processes that contribute to a low-level adaptive response and create barriers to learning. When teachers observe and report at-risk affect or behaviors in their students, unique perspectives and assumptions, explored and blended within the collaborative model, steer the education team toward more comprehensive assessment and more effective and targeted interventions for kids who struggle in school.

School environments offer a complex sensory challenge. The discussion of SMD in this chapter should increase awareness of the physical environmental components of color, sound, proximity, tactile opportunities, social engagement, and the sheer number of visual images that derive from posted displays, as well as the movement and activity of adults and peers in the visual space. The variety of school environments, each with unique sensations to manage, must be considered when children's behavioral responses fail to create an adaptive match to performance demands. Collaboration between teachers and OTs at the level of core instruction will not only benefit those children who struggle to meet the expectations of education, but will also serve a preventive model that supports and enables all children's readiness to learn.

The principles of sensory processing offer a significant and constructive contribution to the development of curricular strategies and methods. Processing through all sensory channels has implications for learning. The near senses (i.e., tactile, vestibular, and proprioceptive) are foundational for self-regulation and movement. Movement and learning are strongly linked. When young children struggle to maintain optimal arousal and learning readiness or to meet the increasingly rigorous demands of the K–3 curriculum, the playful engagement of the body in learning is central to their educational success. The task demands of literacy and mathematical concepts and skills, which may still the body and constrain the partnership of far and near senses, can easily be altered to create a better match for the learning needs of all young children.

Appendix

Common classroom modifications for sensory modulation disorder (SMD): Rationale and effect on adaptive response

SEATING AND POSITIONING

Strategy	Rationale	Benefit and effect on adaptive response
Dynamic cushion	Wedge-shaped: allows child-generated minor movement in linear front to back plane (some bounce) Disc-shaped: allows child-generated variable movement in all planes; heavy work to postural core; can be used on chair or floor	Increases proprioception and thus arousal; suits degree of movement to child; enhances attention; extends work endurance; outlet for sensory-seeking behavior; use on floor to delineate child's space, increasing comfort in group (placing child at periphery can be more tolerable to overresponsive child); increases intensity of sensation
Rocking chair; glider	Child-generated, rhythmic, linear movement	Child adjusts movement intensity to calm or alert; enhances attention; extends work endurance during quiet times (silent reading); delineates space; provides respite when child needs a break
Cube chair; booster seat; armchair	Provides tactile boundaries around child's body	Provides constant, predictable pressure touch for calming (especially if padded); delineates space on floor; increases duration of sensation
Small inner tube	"Cradles" child when seated on floor	Provides constant, predictable pressure touch for calming; child-generated movement as tolerated; delineates space on floor; provides respite
Therapy ball	Can be used as alternative to desk chair; provides child-generated movement in multiple planes; can be used for universal support to whole class. Variations for floor: inflated "animal seat," inflated stool, bolster, peanut-shaped ball	Rock for calming; bounce for alerting; extends work endurance and attention to task; outlet for sensory-seeking behavior; adjusts intensity, frequency, duration

Strategy	Rationale	Benefit and effect on adaptive response
"Uneven" chair	One shorter leg on chair provides for minor rocking	Can be alerting or calming; outlet for sensory-seeking behavior
Beanbag chair; large pillows	Envelops child when seated or provides "crash" pad; child can "burrow" under pillows	Deep pressure touch to multiple body surfaces; calms; burrowing allows "escape" and/or respite Crash pad increases proprioception for organization of behavior; outlet for sensory-seeking behavior; increases intensity
T-stool; rolling chair	Child-generated movement in variable planes and directions	Proprioception from postural core; alerts and/or organizes; extends work endurance and attention to task; outlet for sensory-seeking behavior; adjusts intensity, frequency, duration

ENVIRONMENTAL MODIFICATIONS

Strategy	Rationale	Benefit and effect on adaptive response
Modify walls	Limit decorations and/or hangings to include at least one "neutral" wall; paint with calming colors (blues and/or greens)	Calms visual environment; removes distraction; enhances attention; prevents gradual escalation of arousal
Modify lighting	Turn fluorescent lights down on sunny day; include lamplight; use "daylight" bulbs or full spectrum lighting	Reduces harsh light; calms visual environment; enhances attention; may increase work duration; prevents gradual escalation of arousal; flashing lights may be intolerable to overresponsive child
Modify sound	Provide background music to suit needs of student; provide movement break; provide rhythm; provide warnings of loud sound (fire drill)	Provides calming or alerting auditory sensation Calming: quiet, nature sounds; beat-per-second rhythms; predictable; moderation of teacher voice; "silent clapping" Alerting: loud, variable rhythms; unanticipated sound (clapping or burst of laughter)

Strategy	Rationale	Benefit and effect on adaptive response
Consider furniture	Are children too close? Is there enough space at table? Do chairs fit child? Do chairs make noise when moved on floor? Does furniture leave enough floor space to allow for variable body positions during floor play?	More space "protects" tactile or movement-sensitive child and reduces likelihood of unwanted touching by sensory-seeking child; well-fit chairs provide contact with feet on floor for movement-sensitive child; alternative floor play enhances tactile encounters, pressure to body, natural movement
Designated sensory room	Designed by the OT to include specialized equipment for maximal benefit to children with SPD	Individualized therapy; supervised movement or respite breaks; restores self-regulation and enables ability to reengage in occupational tasks with optimal adaptive response
Seat assignment	Provide placement at periphery; experiment with back or front of classroom; change positions regularly for novelty	Distracted or visually overresponsive child at front; underresponsive child in front to receive instructional cues; novelty for underresponsive child; sensory-seeking child in back to allow for standing, stretching, or movement without disturbing others; experiment for movement-sensitive or touch-sensitive child; slightly separate desk to prevent unanticipated touch or reduce proximity of peers
Study carrel	Modifies child's immediate visual (some sound) environment; limits distraction	Increases focus on immediate task; some respite (*Note:* consider impact on constructivist learning methods. OT and teacher should negotiate regarding other options for supported group encounters.)
Room arrangement	Open space; carpeted space; respite corner; reading "loft"; space for mini-trampoline or rocking board; higher counter for standing work	Room for movement breaks; space for alternative positions to encourage postural and antigravity adjustment for baseline arousal; social engagement; separation when necessary; respite breaks
Modify storage	Cover or enclose extraneous materials (book shelves, dress-up clothing; blocks); unify storage containers; consider height of storage to encourage stooping, reaching, stretching	Covering materials removes distraction; unifies visual environment; calms; prevents gradual escalation of arousal Height of storage facilitates proprioception via movement opportunity

WEARABLES

Strategy	Rationale	Benefit and effect on adaptive response
Weighted vest, shoulder "snake" or lap pad; weighted backpack	Increases proprioception and deep pressure touch	Calms and/or organizes for self-regulation; increases attention and adaptive response; limits sensory-seeking behavior; weighted backpack can be worn during transition times between classrooms to organize the overresponsive or sensory-seeking child; regulates intensity, duration
Spandex or Lycra clothing; bike shorts; pressure vests	Increases deep pressure touch	Calms and/or organizes for self-regulation; regulates intensity, duration
"Body sock" or Lycra wrap	Increases deep pressure touch; "heavy" (resistive) work	Calms and/or organizes for self-regulation; respite activity; can be incorporated into classroom movement games; social engagement
Hooded sweat-shirt; soft, worn, or all-cotton clothing; seam-less socks; tags removed	Increases warm and/or tolerable touch; hood allows for occasional "escape"	Calms and/or organizes for self-regulation; eliminates sources of nonhabituating tactile sensation that can distract the overrespon-sive child and escalate behavior
Headphones	Provide soothing or alerting sound or no sound; filter or eliminate ambient sound via general noise reduction	Calms, alerts, or organizes for self-regulation; provides respite from multiple sound environments of classroom; increases attention to task; may improve test taking; eliminates source of nonhabituat-ing auditory sensation

MATERIALS

Strategy	Rationale	Benefit and effect on adaptive response
General toys and/or materials	Consider sensory characteristics, including texture, color, sound, weight	Note that weighted toys (heavy balls, weighted blocks, or building bricks) provide increased proprio-ception and "heavy work" for embedded regulatory sensation throughout the day

Strategy	Rationale	Benefit and effect on adaptive response
Fidget toys	Any combination of sensory characteristics: squishy, soft, bumpy, vibrating, bendable, stretchy, smooth and/or hard, scratchy, weighted. Allow anytime access or during "listening" times or transitions	Tailored to sensory needs of child; self-regulation; outlet for sensory-seeking behavior; enables selective attention; prevents child from touching and/or pestering peers (note: to prevent distraction to peers, select quiet toys during listening times); regulates frequency, duration, some intensity
Chewables and other oral options	Chewable bracelets or necklaces, whistles, straws, harmonicas, age-appropriate choices for oral exploration	Allows for self-regulation, attention; provides outlet for oral sensory-seeking (especially for child who chews and/or sucks clothing); provides a source of "heavy work" to specific muscles and joints

Snacks	Flavors:
	    Intense (cinnamon, citrus, salty)
	    Bland (vanilla)
	
	Intense textures: crunchy, chewy
	
	"Heavy work" to muscles of mouth: strong sucking through small straw; thickened liquids (yogurt, milkshake); lollipop; gum
	
	Temperature
		All for self-regulation:
		Alerting
		Calming
		
		Alerting
		
		Organizing
		
		Cold for alerting; warm for calming

Olfactory options	Aroma kits	Assists with self-regulation (calming or alerting); promotes attention
Vibration	Teething toys; pillows; small massagers; stuffed animals	Initially alerting; calming over time
Tactile placemat	Needlepoint grid, sandpaper, tub decals	Place under coloring paper to increase sensory feedback: alerting; can sustain attention to task
Bright placemat	Orange, red, yellow under written work	Alerting; sustains attention
Roller or rocker board under feet; spandex wrap on chair legs	"Fidgets" for the feet	Provides outlet for sensory-seeking behavior; spandex offers heavy work or resistance for self-regulation; regulates frequency, intensity, duration
Velcro tabs	Place on or under edge of desktop: loops for soothing touch, hooks for alerting touch	Assists with self-regulation; provides outlet for sensory-seeking behavior; inconspicuous

Strategy	Rationale	Benefit and effect on adaptive response
Small fans	Handheld as fidget toy; desktop as sound and/or tactile sensation	Assists with self-regulation; alerting; provides "white noise" for masking ambient sound
Sensory bins and tables	Fill with beans, cornmeal, sand, rice, water, bubbles	Assists with self-regulation; provides outlet for sensory-seeking behavior; can gradually desensitize child to touch, depending on material. (*Note:* slimy textures are often rejected by the overresponsive child; lightweight materials [rice] can overstimulate a child and create disorganized behavior) *Do not force participation*

ROUTINE

Strategy	Rationale	Benefit and effect on adaptive response
Early arrival or dismissal	Enables packing or unpacking before group arrives	Reduces likelihood of unwanted physical contact or "chaotic" movement; enables selective attention to arrival and/or dismissal routine; provides a better start and end to the day
Movement breaks	Embed regularly into daily routine and learning activities; allow extra as needed	Excellent for self-regulation of all children; enhances learning via the movement–learning link
Special assignments	Additional movement breaks (bring attendance to office; hand out or collect papers; stack books; erase board; carry materials bin while walking in line; be door holder, note taker, stopwatch manager)	Creates embedded proprioception and movement for self-regulation; provides respite; provides outlet for sensory-seeking behavior; provides protection from unwanted sensation; promotes self-esteem and confidence
Daily schedule	Predictable or novel, depending on child's needs	Predictable for overresponsive child; novelty for underresponsive or sensory-seeking child
Visual schedule	Aids predictability of daily events and transitions	Reduces anticipatory anxiety and hypervigilance; facilitates work duration when breaks are known

Strategy	Rationale	Benefit and effect on adaptive response
Timers	Aid predictability of work session or end of break	Reduces anticipatory anxiety; facilitates work duration
		Visual timer for child who processes best through visual channel

6

The Knowledge-Sharing Team in Action

Our journey together has carried us into domains of occupational perform-ance that may not readily or fully find their place in the development of pol-icy, in the planning of the academic curriculum, or in the consideration of task demands as they have an impact on the educational outcome of the young child in school. Yet, the old masters of theory, Rousseau, Dewey, Piaget, and Vygotsky honored children's natural instincts to learn, along with active participation in the social and academic environment. In the acquisi-tion of knowledge, they valued the means and were wary of any methodolo-gies that suppress children's abundant experimental tendencies and draw them too quickly beyond their own place of readiness. It is not that the work of the child cannot be steeped in academic objective or that expectations are not in advance of capacity. Indeed, Vygotsky's zone of proximal development (ZPD) assumes that learning *awakens* development and that teaching is ori-ented toward the child's *tomorrow* (Del Río & Álvarez, 2007).

For the young child, however, natural instincts demand an engaged body and intuitively draw on an ideal partnership in the movement–learning link. Modern educators are insightful about this link, although policy deci-sions have, to varying degrees, eliminated recess, play, PE, art, and music; stilled little bodies; and recruited little hands for the more exacting tasks of learning and literacy. From my perspective, there is a theme in a wider resist-ance to the compression of the early childhood curriculum. The more cere-bral the expectations become for young children, the more the body is restrained. With this observation, the occupational therapist (OT) is poised to enter the educational dialogue from an advocacy of the many contributors to occupational performance, particularly of movement as both the mediator and expression of performance foundations and as a powerful neural partner to learning, learning readiness, and adaptive engagement in the environ-ments and tasks of school.

THE CHANGING RELATIONSHIP
BETWEEN TEACHERS AND OCCUPATIONAL THERAPISTS

As education team members are called toward schoolwide screening, cooperation in the identification of at-risk students, and dynamic assessment of performance barriers in the natural environments of school, a mutual understanding of common theoretical influences, applied perspectives, and professional worldviews will complete the conversation of their collaborative efforts toward new best practices in primary education. School-based OTs will provide their best service to children with disabilities and developmental delays when they appreciate the foundations and rationale for the instructional strategies they may seek to modify. They will better understand the child's present levels of performance when they can identify the principal cognitive, academic, linguistic, and attentional demands of tasks that challenge optimal engagement and successful outcome.

Teachers will more readily adapt instructional methods and provide for the needs of all children at the levels of universal and targeted interventions when they can more effectively judge the sensory and motor components of environment and task and incorporate this knowledge for peak learning and for the prevention of academic dysfunction. How does this happen in the real world? Education team members teach each other and learn from each other for the benefit of children. They collaborate *before* the breakdown of occupational performance and bring to the table a heightened awareness of the influence of all domains of development and learning. They mutually view children as dynamic little systems whose interactions with environment and task and the ability to benefit from the scaffolding of others contribute to no less than the plasticity of the growing brain itself. They inform each other of the various task components that they recognize through the lenses of their own unique expertise and share their knowledge as if the success of every child depended on it.

COLLABORATION AT ALL LEVELS

Current educational philosophy demands evidence-based practice, and the burgeoning of rigorous research proffers a vast resource for policymakers in the halls of Congress and for administrators in the halls of schools. The conclusions of research, in the form of stated implications, reciprocally influence practice in the classroom. What a young child is capable of demonstrating cognitively or linguistically may tax a developing motor system or challenge beyond capacity the self-regulatory stability that makes learning possible and natural. This is precisely why we seek *collaborative* rather than solely *consultative* relationships, which may imply expert–novice interaction and fail to nurture the two-way conversations that fully inform the professional team. The research of all school-based professionals, including teachers and OTs, physical therapists, speech and language pathologists, psychologists, and others, can comprehensively address the balance of student, environment, and task and enhance the fruits of collaboration as policy is drawn and as professional training curricula are designed and delivered. The conversation must be broadened to include parents and pre-K educators because the single consideration to postpone explicit handwriting instruction, for example, will filter downward in effect toward the earlier educational environments.

The most effective curriculum committees of local school districts will vet the perspectives of all members of the education team who represent a considerable well of experience and knowledge and whose collaborations will inform the decision-making process as materials and programs are adopted. At the district and school levels, collaborative opportunities are embedded in the calendar and allow time for professionals to share expertise in the form of in-house, in-service trainings and presentations through partnerships with community experts and university faculty. Team-taught staff development trainings offer a diverse array of perspectives when presented by teacher and OT, psychologist and teacher, or OT and speech-language pathologist. Broad topics, such as behavior or writing process, are comprehensively served with this transdisciplinary approach to training and provide an excellent opportunity for knowledge sharing.

School-based education teams have the most immediate opportunity for sharing and planning and the most immediate effect on the daily occupational performance of children based on present circumstances and real encounters. Educators and specialists are experimenting with collaborative and knowledge-sharing intervention models, including strategic instructional teaming by general and special educators or teachers and therapists. Instruction and interventions are modeled via in-class therapy sessions and modified service delivery models that suspend direct therapy intervention at regular intervals to free time for team collaboration. However they are designed, the regular and deliberate collaborations of the entire team are the initial line of defense in the prevention of performance breakdowns when applied to all tiers of a multi-tiered educational model. They form the foundation in the development of interventions and are crucial to successful program modification and student progress monitoring. They mutually appraise environment and task demand and scrutinize instructional strategies for effect on all domains of learning. They have as their goal the successful educational outcome of all children, with due reference to the cognitive, linguistic, sensory, motor, attentional, and self-regulatory processes of the child in the primary grades.

RESTRUCTURING THE
COLLABORATIONS OF THE EDUCATION TEAM

In the transactional model of human ability embraced by Haywood and Lidz (2007), there is a difference between intelligence and cognition. Intelligence originates in genetic endowment and is modestly modifiable with effort. Cognition is acquired and can be modified, unlearned, or relearned. It includes the *processes* of learning, rather than solely the qualities of the learner, and refers to habits, thinking modes, problem-solving approaches, motives, and attitudes, as well as natural abilities. School achievement is further influenced by *nonintellective* variables that might include socioeconomic status, experience, and temperament. In fact, although measured IQ is strongly correlated with the child's school achievement, nearly half of the variance in achievement is associated with variables *other than* IQ.

In the preceding chapters, the understanding of student factors, environmental components, and task demands that also bear on the occupational performance of children in the primary grades have been discussed. Restructuring the collaborations of the education team to systematically address these three components of performance will serve as an incentive to align the theoretical foundations of education professions, include a broader perspective in current evaluation procedures, and create a framework for an all-systems approach to planning and intervention. At the level of core instruction, whether participating in a policy or curriculum meeting or planning strategies for the classroom, education teams should ask themselves a series of questions.

- What are the age range and gender distribution of the classroom and how do instructional strategies address them (e.g., the developmental range in kindergarten, boys and girls in the movement–learning link)?

- Does the adopted curriculum allow for individualization?

- Do we need to consider alternative curricular programs (e.g., vertical handwriting style)?

- How does the physical environment of the classroom influence arousal, attention, sensory processing ability, postural support and movement potential (e.g., color, lighting, uniform storage, gender differences of space per child, visual and auditory elements, alternative seating and positioning, location of technology, alerting and calming elements)?

- Do children's chairs face toward the teacher during explicit instruction or demonstration?

- What kinds of attention bridges are typically used (e.g., raised voice, flashing lights, auditory chime)?

- Do the environment and schedule offer respite (e.g., quiet corner, movement breaks)?

- How does the pace and sequence of the daily schedule support optimal adaptive response (e.g., math after recess, reading after PE)?
- What are the sensory and motor loads of planned instructional tasks?
- How many ways can grade-level expectations be met, other than with desk-bound, paper and pencil activities (e.g., music and rhythm, movement, drama, story telling, haptic exercises)?
- Is learning through far senses and near senses balanced in the classroom?
- How can the child's body be recruited in the movement–learning link?
- What are the *combined* implications of research, and how do they influence the timing, sequence, and methods of instruction?
- How do we integrate the curriculum *and* attend to the automaticity of foundational skills and abilities?
- How can we address the foundations of literacy while waiting for the explicit introduction of handwriting?
- How can we introduce the allographic elements and graphic motor patterns while waiting for the explicit introduction of handwriting?
- How do we relieve the stress that derives from a mismatch between curriculum and developmental readiness at the level of core instruction (further complicated by gender, socioeconomic factors, and waiting time)?
- Is a self-selected curriculum available through play? Does play encourage divergent thinking? Are play and center time distinct?
- How do we engage the entire education team in preventive collaborative efforts for both planning and progress monitoring?
- How can we move toward dynamic assessment?

At the level of targeted intervention, the list of questions becomes more specific.

Student factors

- In which academic domains is the child at risk?
- Which cognitive variables appear to interfere with learning (e.g., memory, attention)?
- Which nonintellective variables influence occupational performance (e.g., arousal, transitions, motor proficiency, response to sensory-rich elements [i.e., tactile, vestibular, proprioceptive])?
- Has the child established a hand preference?
- Does prehension support refined pencil use?
- Does the child show readiness in visual-motor integration skills?

- Do speed and legibility support the handwriting process?
- How mature are the language skills that underlie the writing process (e.g., phonemic awareness, RAN, orthographic awareness)?
- Is the child responsive to all instructional cues (e.g., visual and gestural, auditory and oral, peer transition, written)?
- What are the child's typical self-regulatory strategies (e.g., metacognitive, movement, fidgeting, vocal, private speech, self-isolation), and how effective are they?
- Are responses adaptive (i.e., matched to the demands of environment and task)?
- How effective is posture when seated at a table?
- Can the child maintain learning readiness when in close proximity to peers? In extended periods of quiet or concentrated work? During transitions? When the classroom noise escalates? When engaged in active or non–rule-bound movement activities? When the activity is loaded with an identifiable sensory stimulant (e.g., tactile or sound)? When a sensory event is unpredicted? When plans or routines are changed? In all school environments?
- Do behavioral responses interfere with peer social engagement?
- Can the child readily approach and execute a novel or sequenced motor task?

Environmental components
- Is there an environmental barrier to student performance?
- Does the child's behavior or response *differ* in adaptiveness among the various environments of school (e.g., playground, gymnasium, music room, cafeteria, hallways, circle time)?
- Does adaptive response differ significantly with individual or group activity?
- Does space to child ratio influence behavior or performance (e.g., number of children per table, number of children at centers)?
- Does the environment encourage or restrict movement (e.g., floor space, alternative seating)?
- Does the visual environment distract the child?
- Is the child able to filter the ambient noise of the environment?
- Does behavior tend to escalate with time of day or other variables?
- Is adopted curriculum a good fit, or is alternative instruction necessary?
- Does behavior or adaptive response change significantly with instructional approach? (e.g., implicit versus explicit, didactic versus constructivist)?

- Does behavior or adaptive response change significantly in the different classroom centers?
- Can the child manage behavior during waiting time?
- Are table and chairs a good fit?
- Are adapted materials available for children who struggle with tool use?
- How do schedule and pace influence performance?
- Where, when, and under what circumstances is the child *most* productive and successful?

Task demands

- Do task demands create a barrier to student performance?
- Does the task offer the appropriate challenge for every child?
- What are the sensory components of a challenging task?
- What are the motor requirements of the task?
- What is the linguistic or other cognitive load of the task?
- What are the challenges to working memory?
- What are the attentional requirements (e.g., selective, sustained, need to ignore distraction, need to alternate attention between concurrent tasks)?
- What are the combinatory elements of the task (e.g., ortho-motor, visual-motor)?
- How does performance change with writing mode (e.g., manuscript, cursive, keyboarding)?
- Does performance differ when drawing or writing?
- Does writing performance change significantly with copy, dictation, or composition?
- Does spelling performance differ significantly when oral or written?
- Has automaticity developed for foundational skills?
- How much stillness of body does the task require? How long is the child sitting?
- How are arousal and adaptive response modified by frequency, intensity, and duration of movement or other sensation?
- Which elements of scaffolding are most effective in improving task performance (e.g., leading questions, gestural or other physical cues, demonstration)?
- How does the challenging task *interact* with student factors and environment?
- How much *prevention* is afforded through an effective balance of the three components?

Many more prompts will be added by the unique education team, and the list will undoubtedly change with child age, grade, individual differences, and with the professional backgrounds of the team contributors. At the level of intense intervention (special education), standardized testing will be informative of student factors in the form of *completed* development. Attention to the interactions of student, environment, and task, and progress toward supplemental dynamic assessment will, however, also offer an effective bridge to *potential* development, intervention, and instructional modifications that draw out a child's best performance.

STUDENT–ENVIRONMENT–TASK
AND THE MOVEMENT–LEARNING LINK

In Chapter 4, "When Little Hands Write," handwriting's place in the writing process; its relationship to reading, spelling, and drawing; and the underlying motor proficiencies that support its successful production were reviewed. In this chapter, as the development of a prevention frame of mind is addressed, writing is used as an example and the adjustment of task demand in the alignment of student achievement and learning standards is reviewed.

This chapter adds to the teacher toolbox yet another starter kit for the generation of initial and supplemental instructional activities that draw children toward essential academic learning requirements and grade-level expectations in ways that mitigate stress, liberate the child's cognitive and self-regulatory resources, and naturally profit from the movement–learning link. I am certain that your own education teams already have or will readily fashion countless extraordinary and imaginative ideas toward this end and for every subject area. The point is to plan broadly and to embed movement wherever possible for the enhancement of learning.

"WRITING" WITHOUT WRITING

Stabilizing the allograph

- Post alphabet letters with numbered arrows. Post at eye level those letters that are currently introduced so that children might be enticed to finger trace them if so inclined.
- Play tic-tac-toe with magnetic letters or numbers.
- Tell children to stand up, clap, hop, or touch their toes when the target letter is visually or orally presented.
- Play Red Light, Green Light with letters. Children advance when the target letter is flashed.
- Shape and position bodies to form letters. To draw attention to detail, also have children demonstrate each "stroke" separately with their bodies or arms.

- Play Musical Chairs. Children sit when a targeted letter surfaces in a stack of alphabet cards that are flashed by the teacher or a peer.
- Treasure hunt for three-dimensional letters or numbers hidden in the classroom.
- Identify letters haptically.
- Complete a letter puzzle with eyes closed.
- Construct giant letters with blocks.
- Play Which Direction? Children point or hop and turn their bodies in the correct direction for *b* or *d, p* or *q.*
- Engage children in sequencing so that they perform the correct movement sequence when the model is displayed (e.g., *A* = clap, *B* = stomp, *AB* = clap and stomp).
- Play Concentration with alphabet cards.
- Verbalize displayed letter combinations after a model is removed.
- Play What Am I? Tape a letter to a child's back. Have him or her ask the class a series of yes or no questions until the letter is identified (e.g., "Am I lowercase?" "Do I have a curve?" "Do I dive below the foot line?").
- Ask children for a quick verbal identification of upper case and lowercase when alphabet cards are flashed.
- Play Tall, Small, or Diver? Show children a lowercase alphabet card. Have them call out whether the letter is tall (b, d, f, h, k, l, t), small (a, e, i, m, n, o, s), or diver (g, j, p, q, y).
- Increase the complexity and memory component of Tall, Small, or Diver? by asking children to visualize and name a tall letter, small letter, or diver letter. Or tell them a letter (no visual model) and have them say "tall," "small," or "diver." Eventually say a word and have the children call out the sequence (e.g., "pat" = diver, small, tall).
- Ask children for a quick identification of partially completed letters (e.g., Λ = A). Say what's missing.
- Ask children for a quick identification of letters turned sideways or upside-down.
- Find hidden letters in a design or picture
- Ask children for a quick sort of capitals from lowercase forms.
- Do a quick match of manuscript with cursive counterpart using cards or three-dimensional letters.
- Use letter stamps or letter punches.

Stabilizing the graphic motor pattern

- Increase complexity of air writing by having children isolate and produce only the stroke that comes first, second, or third or last.

- Air write with elbow or toes.
- Sensory write in sand, shaving cream, or clay trays (resistance enhances proprioception).
- Play The Writing Train. Children visualize a giant letter on the floor; one group "chugs along" in correct direction to form the first stroke, then additional groups form remaining strokes in the correct direction.
- Create art projects that incorporate correct directional strokes (e.g., apples on a tree or pumpkins on a fence for counterclockwise circles)
- Create yarn letters by having children glue yarn over letters on paper. First, "write" the letter with glue in correct direction and stroke sequence. Then use separate lengths of yarn for each separate stroke.
- Create collage letters by having children tear small pieces of construction paper and glue them to form a letter in the correct stroke direction and sequence.
- Create block letters by having children form a letter by lining large or small blocks in the correct direction and sequence.
- Play Where's the Arrow? Children add the directional arrows to letters provided on a page or whiteboard.
- Play Follow the Arrows. The teacher places only the arrows on the whiteboard in the correct direction and sequence. Children guess the letter.
- Play Head or Belt. The teacher names or shows a letter, and the children touch their head or waist to indicate where the letter starts.
- Play Show Me the Way. The teacher points to one of the lines of a letter, and the children use their fingers to point up, down, left, or right to indicate the starting direction of the stroke.
- Play Silly Sounds in which children provide the "sound of a stroke." For example, children provide a descending vocalization every time the teacher forms a stroke from top to bottom. Alternatively use musical instruments to supply the sounds (e.g., xylophone, flute, kazoo).
- Children take turns to recall and name all lowercase letters that start at the headline (e.g., *b, h, k, l, t*). Name those letters that have a curve or have a horizontal or diagonal stroke (similar to "Tall, Small, or Diver?").
- Play Letter, Sound, Stroke. The first child names a letter, the second child names the letter sound, and the third child writes the letter in the air.
- Model phonemic segmentation and strokes. The teacher writes a word on the whiteboard; erases a beginning or end letter; then air writes the letter to be substituted. The children name the new word.

- Play Phoneme to Grapheme. The teacher pronounces the letter sound, and the children air write or form body letters for the corresponding grapheme. The teacher can reverse the learning task by air writing the letter and having the children produce the sound.

Word spacing

- A sentence is built as children stand with word cards. The children act as spacers by standing between words and stretching their arms to push words apart.
- Overspace magnetic words or word cards.
- Play Teacher's Mistake. Have children correct the teacher's unspaced sentence on the board.
- Play Clap the Space. Children clap to cue the teacher to space as he or she writes a sentence on the whiteboard (or exchange clapping for stomping, standing, sitting, turning, or hopping).

Line orientation

- Create art projects with objects on a baseline (e.g., cut out and glue cars on a road, stamp shapes on a baseline).
- Place magnetic letters or words on a baseline drawn on the whiteboard.
- Place letter stamps correctly between two or three lines on paper.
- Use letter tiles on paper to space and orient to lines. Use two blank tiles for word spacing.
- Play Who's Getting Tired? The teacher incorrectly places magnetic letters within lines. The children identify and correctly place the letters that are not resting on the baseline.
- Children balance on a 1- to 2-inch high balance beam (or on a line on the floor) as they form letters with their body, demonstrating careful attention to baseline orientation.
- Play Out to Dry. Stretch a clothesline or string across the whiteboard. Children use clips or clothespins to attach *tall* letters above the line and *diver* letters below the line.

Spelling

- Use magnetic letters on metal cookie sheets to create Elkonin Boxes (squares on whiteboard or paper, each containing a separate syllable or a single phoneme of a word).
- Stretch arms horizontally when the teacher pronounces a long vowel and hang arms at sides for short vowel.
- Children (holding letter cards) stand side by side to form a consonant-vowel-consonant (CVC) word. They replace each other to manipulate onset and rime. (*Onset* is the portion of a syllable that

precedes its vowel [e.g., **drop**]. Rime contains the syllable's vowel and the consonants that follow [e.g., d**rop**]).

- Play Concentration with letter combinations (e.g., *ea, ie, er*).
- Set high-frequency word spellings to music.
- Tape word cards to beanbags. Sort (toss) correctly spelled words from incorrectly spelled words. (Caution: This game may not be appropriate for children with learning disabilities who may retain "plausible errors.")
- Spell words while bouncing on therapy balls to increase fluency and enhance memory.

Idea generation

- Play beanbag toss in which the catcher offers the next sentence in a group story and then tosses the beanbag to the next student.
- Have one student act out an animal, and then have a team member offer a sentence about it.
- Group one orally composes a story, and group two illustrates the story on large paper (on a vertical surface or on the floor)
- Group one collects objects or props from the classroom and places them in a sequence. Group two then composes a story that includes the props in correct sequence (the teacher can transcribe).
- The teacher composes a story, leaving out the nouns, and the children add nouns after haptically identifying an object in their hand.
- Children literally build a story from blocks labeled with words or phrases (e.g., *Once upon a time, there was a, cat, mouse, bird*). Blocks can be labeled on all sides, similar to dice.
- Each child is given a word or phrase card. The class then builds a story by arranging peers in the desired sequence in front of the class. Revisions can be made by rearranging classmates.

Word usage

- Boys stand when *he, him,* or *his* is heard in a sentence; girls stand for *she, her,* or *hers*.
- Perform the action of verbs.
- Match correct singular or plural word card to single- or multiple-object group.

Punctuation

- The teacher reads large font sentences or story (so that children can see punctuation marks in print). Children add silly motions and sounds for each punctuation mark as story is read.

With the principles of the student–environment–task balance in mind and attention to the movement–learning link, education teams can register a catalog of new or alternative strategies that are perfectly suited to the multiple developmental needs of young students and recruit the active qualities that characterize their natural learning efforts. Pencils will be idle for longer periods of time, and little hands will be raised in playful engagement within the literacy curriculum.

ASSESSMENT AND STUDENT–ENVIRONMENT–TASK

Despite the most careful planning of environmental components and task demands, some children (fewer, it is anticipated) will continue to struggle to meet the performance expectations for grade, and individualized assessment will be recommended by the school's referral team. Standardized testing is likely to be a component of the process, although school specialists, including psychologists and therapists, are increasingly thinking beyond classification provided by normative assessment results and toward greater collaboration regarding potential interventions.

In a broad approach to primary educational assessment, the team's efforts to balance the components of occupational performance will contribute significantly to amelioration of many factors that may inadvertently place some children at risk. The team that is already thinking in terms of the mutual influences of student, environment, and task may well consider a form of dynamic assessment as a complement to standardized testing and as having additional potential to advance the critical identification of both barriers and contributors to successful performance outcome.

Dynamic assessment supplements and extends understanding by comparing children to changes in their own performance as moderated by intensity, frequency, and type of instruction, as well as with modifications to context and task. The approach is sometimes criticized as time consuming, as it taxes the full schedules and defined timelines of evaluation teams. Under current pull-out assessment procedures, assuming the responsibility for several sessions of strategy trials might certainly become unwieldy for professionals who also maintain an active caseload of direct intervention services. Indeed, the adoption of dynamic assessment would require a creative rethinking of the roles and service models for school-based therapists and school psychologists. Although this assessment approach has not yet been widely embraced in educational centers, it is worthy of a thorough review of both its drawbacks and potential strengths in addressing the multiple variables of occupational performance for children in the primary grades.

CONCLUSION

The decade of the brain raised consciousness of the integration of neural structures in learning and the interdependence of learning domains. This recent awareness has come full circle as education teams begin to implement strategies that more systematically grant due consideration to the same inter-relatedness of factors *outside* the brain that have equally substantial influence on learning itself.

In crossing paths in the educational environment, teachers and OTs have so much to share—common theoretical foundations, influences that mutually frame their professional goals, and unique knowledge that contributes to an inclusive picture of the young child in school. Consideration of the terms of developmentally appropriate practice will be retained as the team filters the curriculum through the influences of environmental components and task demand. Stress factors will be reduced or eliminated as education teams share their knowledge to collaborate on the pace and timing of instruction, alternative instructional strategies based on the combined components of all developmental domains, the need for space and movement, the relative meaning of *appropriate challenge*, the wide developmental range of the youngest learners, and the various needs of boys and girls. We have much to share regarding the readiness of children for the tasks of school and the readiness of schools to receive all children.

It is not difficult to imagine that education teams might have their own ZPD and scaffold new understandings for each other in the best interest of children. By collaborating at all levels, we move beyond the completed development of our own professional expertise and into the zone of potential development that can only derive from knowledge-sharing between competent others in the working environment. We do not share knowledge simply because we have interesting things to say, but because research has confirmed the intimate links between educational outcome and occupational performance, between movement and cognition, between executive and sensory self-regulation, and between sensory-based arousal and attention to task. We become better prepared to plan best practice strategies and can most strategically intervene to ensure that student factors, environmental components, and task demands are in balance. Most importantly, children are the beneficiaries as we acknowledge the embodied processes of learning and release the playful dispositions and natural energies of our youngest learners in school.

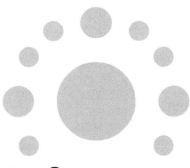

References

Abbott, R.D., & Berninger, V.W. (1993). Structural equation modeling of relationships among developmental skills and writing skills in primary- and intermediate-grade writers. *Journal of Educational Psychology, 85*(3), 478–508.

Ackerman, D.J., & Barnett, W.S. (2005, March). *Prepared for kindergarten: What does "readiness" mean?* NIEER Policy Report. New Brunswick, NJ: National Institute for Early Education Research.

Adi-Japha, E., & Freeman, N.H. (2001). Development of differentiation between writing and drawing systems. *Developmental Psychology, 37,* 101–114.

Ahn, R.R., Miller, L.J., Milberger, S., & McIntosh, D.N. (2004). Prevalence of parents' perceptions of sensory processing disorders among kindergarten children. *The American Journal of Occupational Therapy, 58*(3), 287–293.

American Occupational Therapy Association. (2006). Workforce trends in occupational therapy. Retrieved December 20, 2007, from http://www.aota.org/search.aspx?SearchPhrase=workforce+trends

American Occupational Therapy Association. (2008). *Occupational therapy practice framework: Domain and process* (2nd ed.). Bethesda, MD: Author.

Annett, M. (1998). The stability of handedness. In K.J. Connolly (Ed.), *The psychobiology of the hand* (pp. 63–76). London: Mac Keith Press.

Apel, K., Wolter, J.A., & Masterson, J.J. (2006). Effects of phonotactic and orthotactic probabilities during fast mapping on 5-year-olds' learning to spell. *Developmental Neuropsychology, 29*(1), 21–42.

Armstrong, D.F., Stokoe, W.C., & Wilcox, S.E. (1995). *Gesture and the nature of language*. Cambridge, England: Cambridge University Press.

Arnheim, R. (1974). *Art and visual perception: A psychology of the creative eye*. (50th anniversary printing). Berkeley, CA: University of California Press.

Arnold, E.M., Goldston, D.B., Walsh, A.K., Reboussin, B.A., Daniel, S.S., Hickman, E., et al. (2005). Severity of emotional and behavioral problems among poor and typical readers. *Journal of Abnormal Child Psychology, 33*(2), 205–217.

Ayres, A.J. (1972). *Sensory integration and learning disorders*. Los Angeles: Western Psychological Services.

Bakhurst, D. (2007). Vygotsky's demons. In H. Daniels, M. Cole, & J.V. Wertsch (Eds.), *The Cambridge companion to Vygotsky* (pp. 50–76). New York: Cambridge University Press.

Barnhart, R.C., Davenport, M.J., Epps, S.B., & Nordquist, V.M. (2003). Developmental coordination disorder. *Physical Therapy, 83*(8), 722–731

Baumer, S., Ferholt, B., & Lecusay, R. (2005). Promoting narrative competence through adult–child joint pretense: Lessons from the Scandinavian educational practice of playworld. *Cognitive Development, 20*, 576–590.

Baumgartner, T., Willi, M., & Jäncke, L. (2007). Modulation of corticospinal activity by strong emotions evoked by pictures and classical music: A transcranial magnetic stimulation study. *NeuroReport, 18*(3), 261–265. Retrieved April 9, 2009, from http://www.brainmusic.org/EducationalActivitiesFolder/Baumgartner_emotion2007.pdf

Beery, K.E., & Beery, N.A. (2004). *The Beery-Buktenica Developmental Test of Visual Motor-Integration: Administration, scoring, and teaching manual* (5th ed.). Minneapolis: Pearson.

Beitchman, J. (2005). Language development and its impact on children's psychosocial and emotional development. *Encyclopedia on early childhood development*. Retrieved June 5, 2007, from http://www.child-encyclopedia.com/documents/BeitchmanANGxp.pdf

Bergen, D. (2002). The role of pretend play in children's cognitive development. *Early Childhood Research & Practice, 4*(1). Retrieved August 12, 2008, from http://ecrp.uiuc.edu/v4n1/bergen.html

Berk, L.E. (2001). *Awakening children's minds: How parents and teachers can make a difference*. New York: Oxford University Press.

Berninger, V.W. (1999). Coordinating transcription and text generation in working memory during composing: Automatic and constructive processes. *Learning Disability Quarterly, 22*(2), 99–112.

Berninger, V.W. (2004). Understanding the "graphia" in developmental dysgraphia: A developmental neuropsychological perspective for disorders in producing written language. In D. Dewey & D.E. Tupper (Eds.), *Developmental motor disorders: A neuropsychological perspective* (pp. 328–350). New York: Guilford Press.

Berninger, V.W., Abbott, R.D., Abbott, S.P., Graham, S., & Richards, T. (2002). Writing and reading: Connections between language by hand and language by eye. *Journal of Learning Disabilities, 35*(1), 39–57.

Berninger, V.W., Abbott, R.D., Jones, J., Wolf, B.J., Gould, L., Anderson-Youngstrom, M., et al. (2006). Early development of language by hand: Composing, reading, listening, and speaking connections; three letter-writing modes; and fast mapping in spelling. *Developmental Neuropsychology, 29*(1), 61–92.

Berninger, V.W., Vaughan, K.B., Abbott, R.D., Abbott, S.P., Rogan, L.W., Brooks, A., et al. (1997). Treatment of handwriting problems in beginning writers: Transfer from handwriting to composition. *Journal of Educational Psychology, 89*(4), 652–666.

Bowers, P.G., & Ishaik, G. (2003). RAN's contribution to understanding reading disabilities. In H.L. Swanson, K.R. Harris, & S. Graham (Eds.), *Handbook of learning disabilities* (pp. 140–157). New York: Guilford Press.

Braswell, G.S., & Rosengren, K.K. (2000). Decreasing variability in the development of graphic production. *International Journal of Behavioural Development, 24*(2), 153–166.

Bredekamp, S. (2004). Play and school readiness. In E.F. Zigler, D.G. Singer, & S.J. Bishop-Josef (Eds.), *Children's play: The roots of reading* (pp. 159–174). Washington, DC: Zero to Three Press.

Bredekamp, S., & Copple, C. (Eds.). (1997). *Developmentally appropriate practice in early childhood programs* (Rev. ed.). Washington, DC: National Association for the Education of Young Children.

Brenneman, K., Massey, C., Machado, S.F., & Gelman, R. (1996). Young children's plans differ for writing and drawing. *Cognitive Development, 11*, 397–419.

Brooks, J.G., & Brooks, M.G. (2001). *In search of understanding: The case for constructivist classrooms* (2nd ed.). Upper Saddle River, NJ: Prentice Hall.

Burton, A.W., & Dancisak, M.J. (2000). Grip form and graphomotor control in preschool children. *The American Journal of Occupational Therapy, 54*(1), 9–17.

Burts, D.C., Hart, C.H., Charlesworth, R., DeWolf, D.M., Ray, J., Manuel, K., et al. (1993). Developmental appropriateness of kindergarten programs and academic outcomes in first grade. *Journal of Research in Childhood Education, 8*(1), 23–31.

Burts, D.C., Hart, C.H., Charlesworth, R., Fleege, P.O., Mosley, J., & Thomasson, R.H. (1992). Observed activities and stress behaviors of children in developmentally appropriate and inappropriate kindergarten classrooms. *Early Childhood Research Quarterly, 7*, 297–318.

Burts, D.C., Hart, C.H., Charlesworth, R., & Kirk, L. (1990). A comparison of frequencies of stress behaviors observed in kindergarten children in classrooms with developmentally appropriate versus developmentally inappropriate instructional practices. *Early Childhood Research Quarterly, 5*, 407–423.

Bush, G.H.W. (1990). Presidential proclamation 6158. Retrieved April 9, 2009, from http://www.loc.gov/loc/brain/proclaim.html

Campbell, J. (1995). *Understanding John Dewey: Nature and cooperative intelligence.* Chicago: Open Court.

Center on Education Policy. (2006, March). *From the capital to the classroom: Year 4 of the No Child Left Behind Act.* Retrieved October 18, 2007, from

http://www.cep-dc.org/document/docWindow.cfm?fuseaction=docu
ment.viewDocument&documentid=194&documentFormatId=1183

Center on Education Policy. (2007, December). *Choices, changes, and challenges: Curriculum and instruction in the NCLB era.* Retrieved March 18,
2009, from http://www.cep-dc.org/document/docWindow.cfm?fuseaction=
document.viewDocument&documentid=212&documentFormatId=4154

Chafin, S., Roy, M., Gerin, W., & Christenfeld, N. (2004). Music can facilitate blood pressure recovery from stress. *British Journal of Health
Psychology, 9,* 393–403.

Colello, S.M.G. (2001, July). *The role of drawing in children's writing.* Study
presented at Congresso de Leitura do Brasil. English translation retrieved
January 25, 2008, from http://www.hottopos.com/rih6/silvia.htm

Coolahan, K., Fantuzzo, J., Mendez, J., & McDermott, P. (2000). Preschool
peer interactions and readiness to learn: Relationships between classroom peer play and learning behaviors and conduct. *Journal of
Educational Psychology, 92*(3), 458–465.

Cornhill, H., & Case-Smith, J. (1996). Factors that relate to good and poor
handwriting. *The American Journal of Occupational Therapy, 50*(9),
732–739.

Daly, C.J., Kelley, G.T., & Krauss, A. (2003). Relationship between visual-
motor integration and handwriting skills of children in kindergarten: A
modified replication study. *The American Journal of Occupational Therapy,
57*(4), 459–462.

Damrosch, L. (2005). *Jean-Jacques Rousseau: Restless genius.* Boston:
Houghton Mifflin.

Daniels, H. (2007). Pedagogy. In H. Daniels, M. Cole & J.V. Wertsch (Eds.),
The Cambridge companion to Vygotsky (pp. 307–331). New York:
Cambridge University Press.

Daniels, H., Cole, M., & Wertsch, J.V. (Eds.). (2007). *The Cambridge companion to Vygotsky.* New York: Cambridge University Press.

Davies, P.L., & Gavin, W.J. (2007). Validating the diagnosis of sensory processing disorders using EEG technology. *The American Journal of
Occupational Therapy, 61*(2), 176–189.

Del Río, P., & Álvarez, A. (2007). Inside and outside the Zone of Proximal
Development: An ecofunctional reading of Vygotsky. In H. Daniels, M.
Cole & J.V. Wertsch (Eds.), *The Cambridge companion to Vygotsky* (pp.
276–303). New York: Cambridge University Press.

Dennis, J.L., & Swinth, Y. (2001). Pencil grasp and children's handwriting
legibility during different-length writing tasks. *The American Journal of
Occupational Therapy, 55*(2), 175–183.

Denton, P.L., Cope, S., & Moser, C. (2006). The effects of sensorimotor-
based intervention versus therapeutic practice on improving handwriting performance in 6- to 11-year-old children. *American Journal of
Occupational Therapy, 60*(1), 16–27.

DeVries, R., Zan, B., Hildebrandt, R., Edmiaston, R., & Sales, C. (2002). *Developing constructivist early childhood curriculum: Practical principles and activities*. New York: Teachers College Press.

Diamond, A. (2000). Close interrelation of motor development and cognitive development and of the cerebellum and prefrontal cortex. *Child Development, 71*(1), 44–56.

Dunn, W. (2001). The sensations of everyday life: Empirical, theoretical, and pragmatic considerations. *The American Journal of Occupational Therapy, 55*(6), 608–620.

Dwyer, T., Sallis, J.F., Blizzard, L., Lazarus, R., & Dean, K. (2001). Relation of academic performance to physical activity and fitness in children. *Pediatric Exercise Science, 13*, 225–237.

Education for All Handicapped Children Act of 1975, PL 94-142, 20 U.S.C. §§ 1400 *et seq.*

Egan, K. (1997). *The educated mind: How cognitive tools shape our understanding*. Chicago: The University of Chicago Press.

Egan, K. (2005). *An imaginative approach to teaching*. San Francisco: Jossey-Bass.

Eide, B., & Eide, F. (2006). *The mislabeled child: How understanding your child's unique learning style can open the door to success*. New York: Hyperion.

Elbow, P. (2004). Writing first! Putting writing before reading is an effective approach to teaching and learning. *Educational Leadership, 62*(2), 8–13.

Elkind, D. (2007). *The power of play: How spontaneous, imaginative activities lead to happier, healthier children*. Cambridge, MA: Da Capo Press.

Evans, R.I. (1973). *Jean Piaget: The man and his ideas*. New York: Dutton.

Evers, S., Dannert, J., Rödding, D., Rötter, G., & Ringelstein, E.B. (1999). The cerebral haemodynamics of music perception: A transcranial Doppler sonography study. *Brain, 122*, 75–85.

Fagard, J. (1998). Changes in grasping skills and the emergence of bimanual coordination during the first year of life. In K.J. Connolly (Ed.), *The psychobiology of the hand* (pp. 123–143). London: Mac Keith Press.

Fallin, K., Wallinga, C., & Coleman, M. (2001). Helping children cope with stress in the classroom setting. *Childhood Education, 78*(1), 17–24.

Feldman, C.F. (2005). Mimesis: Where play and narrative meet. *Cognitive Development, 20*, 503–513.

Fitzgerald, J., & Shanahan, T. (2000). Reading and writing relations and their development. *Educational Psychologist, 35*(1), 39–50.

Forssberg, H. (1998). The neurophysiology of manual skill development. In K.J. Connolly (Ed.), *The psychobiology of the hand* (pp. 97–122). London: Mac Keith Press.

Fosnot, C.T. (1996). Constructivism: A psychological theory of learning. In C.T. Fosnot (Ed.), *Constructivism: Theory, perspectives, and practice* (pp. 8–33). New York: Teachers College Press.

Gardner, H. (1993). *Frames of mind: The theory of multiple intelligences* (10th anniversary ed.). New York: Basic Books.

Gardner, H. (1999). *Intelligence reframed: Multiple intelligences for the 21st century*. New York: Basic Books.

Gertz, D.S. (2007). *Liebman's neuroanatomy made easy and understandable* (7th ed.). San Antonio, TX: PRO-ED.

Goldberg, M.E., & Hudspeth, A.J. (2000). The vestibular system. In E.R. Kandel, J.H. Schwartz, & M.J. Thomas (Eds.), *Principles of neural science* (4th ed., pp. 801–815). New York: McGraw-Hill.

Golomb, C. (2004). *The child's creation of a pictorial world* (2nd ed.). Mahwah, NJ: Lawrence Erlbaum Associates.

Goyen, T., & Duff, S. (2005). Discriminant validity of the Developmental Test of Visual-Motor Integration in relation to children with handwriting dysfunction. *Australian Occupational Therapy Journal, 52,* 109–115.

Graham, S. (1993/1994, Winter). Are slanted manuscript alphabets superior to the traditional manuscript alphabet? *Childhood Education, 70*(2) 91–95.

Graham, S., Berninger, V.W., Abbott, R.D., Abbott, S.P., & Whitaker, D. (1997). Role of mechanics in composing of elementary school students: A new methodological approach. *Journal of Educational Psychology, 89*(1), 170–182.

Graham, S., Berninger, V., Weintraub, N., & Schafer, W. (1998). Development of handwriting speed and legibility in grades 1–9. *The Journal of Educational Research, 92*(1), 42–52.

Graham, S., & Harris, K.R. (2000). The role of self-regulation and transcription skills in writing and writing development. *Educational Psychologist, 35*(1), 3–12.

Graham, S., Harris, K.R., & Fink, B. (2000). Is handwriting causally related to learning to write? Treatment of handwriting problems in beginning writers. *Journal of Educational Psychology, 92*(4), 620–633.

Graham, S., Weintraub, N., & Berninger, V.W. (1998). The relationship between handwriting style and speed and legibility. *The Journal of Educational Research, 91*(5), 290–296.

Graham, S., Weintraub, N., & Berninger, V. (2001). Which manuscript letters do primary grade children write legibly? *Journal of Educational Psychology, 93*(3), 488–497.

Greer, T., & Lockman, J.J. (1998). Using writing instruments: Invariances in young children and adults. *Child Development, 69*(4), 888–902.

Grissom, J.B. (2005). Physical fitness and academic achievement. *Journal of Exercise Physiology Online, 8*(1), 11–25. Retrieved June 22, 2007, from http://www.asep.org/files/Grissom.pdf

Gurian, M. (2001). *Boys and girls learn differently! A guide for teachers and parents*. San Francisco: Jossey-Bass.

Gurian, M. & Stevens, K. (2005). *The minds of boys: Saving our sons from falling behind in school and life*. San Francisco: Jossey-Bass.

Hadders-Algra, M. (2002). Two distinct forms of minor neurological dysfunction: Perspectives emerging from a review of data of the Groningen Perinatal Project. *Developmental Medicine & Child Neurology, 44*(8), 561–571.

Hart, C.H., Burts, D.C., Durland, M.A., Charlesworth, R., DeWolf, M., & Fleege, P.O. (1998). Stress behaviors and activity type participation of preschoolers in more and less developmentally appropriate classrooms: SES and sex differences. *Journal of Research in Childhood Education, 12*(2), 176–196.

Hayes, J.R., & Flower, L.S. (1980). Identifying the organization of writing processes. In L.W. Gregg, & E.R. Steinberg (Eds.), *Cognitive processes in writing*. Mahwah, NJ: Lawrence Erlbaum Associates.

Haywood, H.C., & Lidz, C.S. (2007). *Dynamic assessment in practice: Clinical and educational applications*. Cambridge, England: Cambridge University Press.

Healy, J.M. (1990). *Endangered minds: Why children don't think and what we can do about it*. New York: Simon & Schuster.

Healy, J.M. (2004). *Your child's growing mind*. New York: Broadway Books.

Henson, K.T. (2001). *Curriculum planning: Integrating multiculturalism, constructivism, and education reform* (2nd ed.). New York: McGraw-Hill.

Hinojosa, J., & Kramer, P. (1999). Developmental perspective: Fundamentals of developmental theory. In P. Kramer & J. Hinojosa (Eds.), *Frames of reference for pediatric occupational therapy* (2nd ed., pp. 3–8). Philadelphia: Lippincott Williams & Wilkins.

Hirsh-Pasek, K., & Golinkoff, R.M. (2003). *Einstein never used flash cards: How our children really learn—and why they need to play more and memorize less*. Emmaus, PA: Rodale Books.

Iacoboni, M. (2003). Understanding intentions through imitation. In S.H. Johnson-Frey (Ed.), *Taking action: Cognitive neuroscience perspectives on intentional acts* (pp. 107–138). Cambridge, MA: The MIT Press.

Individuals with Disabilities Education Improvement Act (IDEA) of 2004, PL 108-446, 20 U.S.C. §§ 1400 *et seq.*

Jeannerod, M. (2003). Simulation of action as a unifying concept for motor cognition. In S.H. Johnson-Frey (Ed.), *Taking action: Cognitive neuroscience perspectives on intentional acts* (pp. 139–163). Cambridge, MA: The MIT Press.

Jenkinson, S. (2001). *The genius of play: Celebrating the spirit of childhood*. Gloucestershire, England: Hawthorn Press.

Jensen, E. (2000a). *Brain-based learning: The new science of teaching and training* (Rev. ed.). San Diego: The Brain Store.

Jensen, E. (2000b). *Learning with the body in mind: The scientific basis for energizers, movement, play, games, and physical education*. Thousand Oaks, CA: Corwin Press.

Jensen, E. (2004). *Brain-compatible strategies* (2nd ed.). San Diego: The Brain Store.

Jones, G.M. (2000). Posture. In E.R. Kandel, J.H. Schwartz, & M.J. Thomas (Eds.), *Principles of neural science* (4th ed., pp. 816–831). New York: McGraw-Hill.

Kagan, S.L., & Kauerz, K. (2007). Reaching for the whole: Integration and alignment in early education policy. In R.C. Pianta, M.J. Cox, & K.L. Snow (Eds.), *School readiness and the transition to kindergarten in the era of accountability* (pp. 11–30). Baltimore: Paul H. Brookes Publishing Co.

Kandel, E.R., & Siegelbaum, S.A. (2000). Overview of synaptic transmission. In E.R. Kandel, J.H. Schwartz, & M.J. Thomas (Eds.), *Principles of neural science* (4th ed., pp. 175–186). New York: McGraw-Hill.

Kimball, J.G. (1999). Sensory integration frame of reference: Theoretical base, function/dysfunction continua, and guide to evaluation. In P. Kramer & J. Hinojosa (Eds.), *Frames of reference for pediatric occupational therapy* (2nd ed., pp. 119–168). Philadelphia: Lippincott Williams & Wilkins.

Kramer, P., & Hinojosa, J. (Eds.). (1999). Developmental perspective: Fundamentals of developmental theory. In *Frames of reference for pediatric occupational therapy* (2nd ed., pp. 3–8). Philadelphia: Lippincott Williams & Wilkins.

Kuhl, D. (1994). *The effect of handwriting style on alphabet recognition.* Paper presented at the Annual Meeting of the American Educational Research Association, April 1, 1994, New Orleans, LA.

Landsmann, L.T., & Karmiloff-Smith, A. (1992). Children's understanding of notations as domains of knowledge versus referential-communicative tools. *Cognitive Development, 7,* 287–300.

LeDoux, J. (2002). *Synaptic self: How our brains become who we are.* New York: Penguin Books.

Lewis, C., Russell, C., & Berridge, D. (1993). When is a mug not a mug? Effects of content, naming, and instructions on children's drawings. *Journal of Experimental Child Psychology, 56,* 291–302.

Liebschner, J. (1992). *A child's work: Freedom and play in Froebel's educational theory and practice.* Cambridge, England: The Lutterworth Press.

Mangeot, S.D., Miller, L.J., McIntosh, D.N., McGrath-Clarke, J., Simon, J., Hagerman, R.J., et al. (2001). Sensory modulation dysfunction in children with attention-deficit-hyperactivity disorder. *Developmental Medicine & Child Neurology, 43,* 399–406.

Manoel, E. de J., & K.J. Connolly. (1998). The development of manual dexterity in young children. In K.J. Connolly (Ed.), *The psychobiology of the hand* (pp. 177–198). London: Mac Keith Press.

Marr, D., & Cermak, S. (2002). Predicting handwriting performance of early elementary students with the Developmental Test of Visual-Motor Integration. *Perceptual and Motor Skills, 95,* 661–669.

Marr, D.M., Windsor, M., & Cermak, S. (2001). Handwriting readiness: Locatives and visuomotor skills in the kindergarten year. *Early Childhood Research & Practice, 3*(1).

Martin, J. (2002). *The education of John Dewey: A biography*. New York: Columbia University Press.

Matuga, J.M. (2004). Situated creative activity: The drawings and private speech of young children. *Creativity Research Journal, 16*(2–3), 267–281.

Maxwell, L.E. (2003). Home and school density effects on elementary school children: The role of spatial density. *Environment and Behavior, 35*(4), 566–578.

McCutchen, D. (2000). Knowledge, processing, and working memory: Implications for a theory of writing. *Educational Psychologist, 35*(1), 13–23.

McMullen, M., Elicker, J., Wang, J., Erdiller, Z., Lee, S., Lin, C., et al. (2005). Comparing beliefs about appropriate practice among early childhood education and care professionals from the U.S., China, Taiwan, Korea and Turkey. *Early Childhood Research Quarterly, 20*, 451–464.

Melillo, R., & Leisman, G. (2004). *Neurobehavioral disorders of childhood: An evolutionary perspective*. New York: Springer Science+Business Media.

Miller, L.J., Anzalone, M.E., Lane, S.J., Cermak, S.A., & Osten, E.T. (2007). Concept evolution in sensory integration: A proposed nosology for diagnosis. *The American Journal of Occupational Therapy, 61*(2), 135–140.

Miller, L.J., Coll, J.R., & Schoen, S.A. (2007). A randomized controlled pilot study of the effectiveness of occupational therapy for children with sensory modulation disorder. *The American Journal of Occupational Therapy, 61*(2), 228–238.

Missiuna, C., Mandich, A.D., Polatajko, H.J., & Malloy-Miller, T. (2001). Cognitive orientation to daily occupational performance (CO-OP): Part I. Theoretical foundations. *Physical & Occupational Therapy in Pediatrics, 20*(2/3), 69–81.

Montessori, M. (1989). *The absorbent mind*. New York: Delta.

Morrow, L.M., & Schickedanz, J.A. (2006). The relationships between sociodramatic play and literacy development. In D.K. Dickinson & S.B. Neuman (Eds.), *Handbook of early literacy research* (Vol. 2, pp. 269–280). New York: Guilford Press.

Mountcastle, V.B. (2005). *The sensory hand: Neural mechanisms of somatic sensation*. Cambridge, MA: Harvard University Press.

Naider-Steinhart, S., & Katz-Leurer, M. (2007). Analysis of proximal and distal muscle activity during handwriting tasks. *The American Journal of Occupational Therapy, 61*(4), 392–398.

Nanof, T. (2007). Capital briefing: Blurring the line between general and special education [Electronic version]. *OT Practice Online, 12*(8), 7.

National Association of State Directors of Special Education, Inc. (2006). *Response to intervention: Policy considerations and implementation*. Alexandria, VA: Author.

National Research Center on Learning Disabilities. (2006). *RTI manual*. Retrieved September 18, 2007, from http://www.nrcld.org/rti_manual/pages/RTIManualIntroduction.pdf

National Research Council. (2000). *How people learn: Brain, mind, experience, and school* (Expanded ed.). Washington, DC: National Academies Press.

National School Readiness Indicators Initiative. (2005, February). *Getting ready: Findings from the National School Readiness Indicators Initiative: A 17-state partnership*. Prepared by Rhode Island KIDS COUNT. Retrieved on May, 6, 2007, from http://www.rikidscount.org/matriarch/documents/Getting%20Ready%20-%20Full%20Report.pdf

No Child Left Behind Act of 2001, PL 107-110, 115 Stat. 1425, 20 U.S.C. §§ 6301 *et seq*.

Noroozian, M., Lotfi, J., Gassemzadeh, H., Emami, H., & Mehrabi, Y. (2002). Academic achievement and learning abilities in left-handers: Guild or gift? *Cortex, 38*(5), 779–785.

Oehler, E., DeKrey, H., Eadry, E., Fogo, J., Lewis, E., Maher, C., & Shilling, A. (2000). The effect of pencil size and shape on the pre-writing skills of kindergartners. *Physical & Occupational Therapy in Pediatrics, 19*(3/4), 53–60.

Office of the High Commissioner for Human Rights, United Nations. (1989). *United Nations Convention on the Rights of the Child: Article 31*. New York. Retrieved November 10, 2006 from http://www.unhchr.ch/html/menu3/b/k2crc.htm

Pehoski, C. (1995). Object manipulation in infants and children. In A. Henderson & C. Pehoski (Eds.), *Hand function in the child: Foundations for remediation* (pp. 136–153). St. Louis: Mosby.

Pfeiffer, B., Henry, A., Miller, S., & Witherell, S. (2008). Effectiveness of Disc 'O' Sit cushions on attention to task in second-grade students with attention difficulties. *The American Journal of Occupational Therapy, 62*(3), 274–281.

Pfeiffer, B., Kinnealey, M., Reed, C., & Herzberg, G. (2005). Sensory modulation and affective disorders in children and adolescents with Asperger's disorder. *The American Journal of Occupational Therapy, 59*(3), 335–345.

Piaget, J. (1975). *The origins of intelligence in children*. New York: International Universities Press.

Pianta, R.C. (2007). Early education in transition. In R.C. Pianta, M.J. Cox, & K.L. Snow (Eds.), *School readiness and the transition to kindergarten in the era of accountability* (pp. 3–10). Baltimore: Paul H. Brookes Publishing Co.

Piek, J.P., & Dyck, M.J. (2004). Sensory-motor deficits in children with developmental coordination disorder, attention deficit hyperactivity disorder and autistic disorder. *Human Movement Science, 23*, 475–488.

Pine, K.J., Lufkin, N., & Messer, D. (2004). More gestures than answers: Children learning about balance. *Developmental Psychology, 40*(6), 1059–1067

Polatajko, H.J., Mandich, A., & Martini, R. (2000). Dynamic performance analysis: A framework for understanding occupational performance. *The American Journal of Occupational Therapy, 54*(1), 65–72.

Pulliam, J.D., & Van Patten, J.J. (1999). *History of education in America* (7th ed.). Upper Saddle River, NJ: Prentice Hall.

Quiroga, V.A.M. (1995). *Occupational therapy: The first 30 years, 1900 to 1930.* Bethesda, MD: American Occupational Therapy Association.

Rapp, B., & Caramazza, A. (1997). From graphemes to abstract letter shapes: Levels of representation in written spelling. *Journal of Experimental Psychology: Human Perception and Performance, 23*(4), 1130–1152.

Rapoport, M., van Reekum, R., & Mayberg, H. (2000). The role of the cerebellum in cognition and behavior: A selective review. *Journal of Neuropsychiatry and Clinical Neurosciences, 12*(2), 193–198.

Reeves, G.D. (2001). Sensory stimulation, sensory integration and the adaptive response. *Sensory Integration Special Interest Section Quarterly, 24*(2), 1–3.

Reeves, G.D., & Cermak, S.A. (2002). Disorders of praxis. In A.C. Bundy, S.J. Lane, & E.A. Murray (Eds.), *Sensory integration theory and practice* (2nd ed., pp. 71–100). Philadelphia: F.A. Davis.

Rosenblum, S., Goldstand, S., & Parush, S. (2006). Relationships among biomechanical ergonomic factors, handwriting product quality, handwriting efficiency, and computerized handwriting process measures in children with and without handwriting difficulties. *The American Journal of Occupational Therapy, 60*(1), 28–39.

Roskos, K., & Christie, J. (2001). Examining the play–literacy interface: A critical review and future directions. *Journal of Early Childhood Literacy, 1*(1), 59–89.

Scheirs, J.G.M. (1990). Relationships between the direction of movements and handedness in children. *Neuropsychologia, 28*(7), 743–748

Schilling, D.L., Washington, K., Billingsley, F.F, & Deitz, J. (2003). Classroom seating for children with attention deficit hyperactivity disorder: Therapy balls versus chairs. *The American Journal of Occupational Therapy, 57*(5), 534–541.

Sharrer, V.W., & Ryan-Wenger, N.A. (2002). School-age children's self-reported stress symptoms. *Pediatric Nursing, 28*(1), 21–27.

Sheridan, S.R. (1997). *Drawing/writing and the new literacy: Where verbal meets visual*. Amherst, MA: Drawing/Writing Publications.

Sousa, D.A. (2001). *How the brain learns: A classroom teacher's guide* (2nd ed.). Thousand Oaks, CA: Corwin Press.

Ste-Marie, D.M., Clark, S.E., Findlay, L.C., & Latimer, A.E. (2004). High levels of contextual interference enhance handwriting skill acquisition. *Journal of Motor Behavior, 36*(1), 115–127.

Stilwell, J.M., & Cermak, S.A. (1995). Perceptual functions of the hand. In A. Henderson & C. Pehoski (Eds.), *Hand function in the child: Foundations for remediation* (pp. 55–80). St Louis: Mosby.

Thelan, E. (1995). Motor development: A new synthesis. *American Psychologist, 50*(2), 79–95.

Thomassen, A.J.W.M., Meulenbroek, R.G.J., & Hoofs, M.P.E. (1992). Economy and anticipation in graphic stroke sequences. *Human Movement Science, 11*, 71–82.

Toglia, J.P. (2005). A dynamic interactional approach to cognitive rehabilitation. In N. Katz (Ed.), *Cognition & occupation across the life span: Models for intervention in occupational therapy* (2nd ed., pp. 29–72). Bethesda, MD: American Occupational Therapy Association.

Turkington, C., & Harris, J.R. (2006). *The encyclopedia of learning disabilities* (2nd ed.). New York: Facts on File.

Tyre, P. (2006, September 11). The new first grade: Too much too soon? *Newsweek, 148*, 34–44.

Tyre, P. (2008). *The trouble with boys: A surprising report card on our sons, their problems at school, and what parents and educators must do*. New York: Crown Publishers.

Unger, J., & Fleischman, S. (2004). Research matters: Is process writing the "write stuff"? *Educational Leadership, 62*(2), 90–91.

van Galen, G.P., Portier, S.J., Smits-Engelsman, B.C.M., & Schomaker, L.R.B. (1993). Neuromotor noise and poor handwriting in children. *Acta Psychologica, 82*, 161–178.

Vernon, S.A., & Ferreiro, E. (1999). Writing development: A neglected variable in the consideration of phonological awareness. *Harvard Educational Review, 69*(4), 395–415.

Viholainen, H., Ahonen, T., Lyytinen, P., Cantell, M., Tolvanen, A., & Lyytinen, H. (2006). Early motor development and later language and reading skills in children at risk of familial dyslexia. *Developmental Medicine & Child Neurology, 48*, 367–373.

Vinter, A. (1999). How meaning modifies drawing behavior in children. *Child Development, 70*(1), 33–49.

Wakely, M.B., Hooper, S.R., de Kruif, R.E.L., & Swartz, C. (2006). Subtypes of written expression in elementary school children: A linguistic-based model. *Developmental Neuropsychology, 29*(1), 125–159.

Washington Office of Superintendent of Public Instruction. (2005). *Washington State learning goals*. Retrieved March 3, 2007, from http://www.k12.wa.us/Curriculuminstruct

Wassenberg, R., Kessels, A.G.H., Kalff, A.C., Hurks, P.P.M., Jolles, J., Feron, F.J.M., et al. (2005). Relation between cognitive and motor performance in 5- to 6-year-old children: Results from a large-scale cross-sectional study. *Child Development, 76*(5), 1092–1103.

Weil, M.J., & Cunningham Amundson, S.J. (1994). Relationship between visuomotor and handwriting skills of children in kindergarten. *The American Journal of Occupational Therapy, 48*(11), 982–988.

Wiedey, L.B., & Lichtenstein, J.M. (1987). *Academic stress in kindergarten children* (Report No. PS 018267). (ERIC Document Reproduction Service No. ED 310865).

Williams, M.S., & Shellenberger, S. (1996). *How does your engine run? A leader's guide to the Alert Program for self-regulation*. Albuquerque, NM: Therapy Works.

Wilson, F.R. (1998). *The hand: How its use shapes the brain, language, and human culture*. New York: Pantheon Books.

Wolfe, P. (2001). *Brain matters: Translating research into classroom practice*. Alexandria, VA: Association for Supervision and Curriculum Development.

Wolfe, P., & Nevills, P. (2004). *Building the reading brain, preK–3*. Thousand Oaks, CA: Corwin Press.

Ziviani, J. (1983). Qualitative changes in dynamic tripod grip between seven and 14 years of age. *Developmental Medicine & Child Neurology, 25*, 778–782.

Ziviani, J., & Elkins, J. (1986). Effect of pencil grip on handwriting speed and legibility. *Educational Review, 38*(3), 247–257.

Zygmunt-Fillwalk, E., & Bilello, T.E. (2005). Parents' victory in reclaiming recess for their children. *Childhood Education, 82*(1), 19–25.

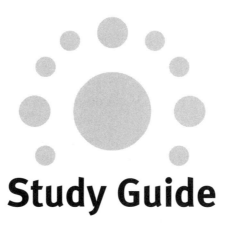

Study Guide

CHAPTER 1
Crossing Paths—Foundations of a Collaborative Prevention Model

1. Discuss the current collaborative model in your school. Do you feel that you recognize the professional influences that bear on the work of your team members? List three ways that knowledge sharing might contribute to the education of the children and the prevention of learning barriers.

2. Discuss three strategies that might enhance collaboration among all members of the education team: administrators, teachers, occupational and physical therapists, speech-language pathologists, psychologists, counselors, parents, and so forth.

3. Arrange for an in-service or seminar on Response to Intervention (RTI) and positive behavior support (PBS). How is your school district moving to implement these models? How might these models change the methods and relationships of the education team?

4. Choose three specific educational activities and discuss the potential student factors, environmental components, and task demands that may influence a student's performance outcome. How might modifying one or more of the components change the student's performance?

5. *Teachers:* Describe to your education team how the theory of constructivism guides your choice of instructional activities, classroom environment, or curriculum projects. *Education team:* Describe 10 academic, linguistic, social-emotional, motor, or sensory components of the described methodology and activities that might challenge some children. How would you address those challenges?

6. What is the chronological age span of entering kindergartners in your school or classroom? *Teachers:* How do the age and maturational ranges of kindergartners influence your own ability to design curricular methods and activities for the group? *Team:* Does the maturational range of

the kindergartners require adaptations to curriculum content or methods? How?

7. *Team:* What are the challenges of maintaining developmentally appropriate practice (DAP) while designing instruction to meet grade-level expectations (GLEs)?

CHAPTER 2
Movement, Occupation, and Learning

1. In introducing the movement–learning link, the author enumerates two principles on which learning professionals should agree. What are they? How does *implicit* learning contribute to the movement–learning link? How is physical activity (e.g., standing, physical fitness) related to the movement–learning link? How does *inactivity* influence the movement–learning link?

2. Name three specific educational activities or academic tasks. What are the motor requirements of each? How might the motor requirements influence performance outcome?

3. *Team collaboration exercise:* Break into small groups of three to five team members. Review your curriculum guide and GLEs. Choose three GLEs and design three new strategies for each, incorporating movement.

4. Consider the pace of the curriculum and your ability to provide *unencumbered practice* for foundational skills. Share strategies that you use to enhance the automaticity of lower level skills in order to free cognitive resources for higher level thinking.

5. Name three ways that you incorporate music and rhythm in the classroom. Can you think of more ways to embed music and rhythm within core subjects such as reading, math, social studies, and science?

6. Discuss the elements of play addressed in Chapter 2. Give examples of play opportunities in your classroom or therapy room that facilitate *convergent* and *divergent* thinking. How do you use play to enhance literacy? Math? Science?

7. Has your school district or grade-level team reduced recess time? Is the change associated with a change in test scores? Think of three alternative strategies (e.g., content integration) that might allow for optimal subject coverage while preserving recess time. Discuss the elimination of recess time as a behavioral consequence. Think of three alternatives to the elimination of recess in the management of student behavior and work production challenges.

8. Discuss the variable movement requirements of boys versus girls. What is the average length of time children spend seated for a single instructional session? Discuss the strategies you use to help students make the transition from an active to a quiet activity. In your school district, how are boys performing academically relative to girls—in math? Language arts? Graduation ratio? Behavioral consequences, such as visits to the principal?

9. Visualize and critique your own classroom or therapy room environment. What are the visual and auditory elements? How does the environment facilitate movement, standing, postural adjustment on the floor? Evaluate space per child. How do these elements influence student attention to task and behavioral self-regulation? What might you change?

CHAPTER 3
Little Hands in School

1. *OTs:* Please answer any questions the team may have regarding the development of hand function and in-hand manipulation. What kinds of fine motor materials do you offer in the classroom or therapy room to enhance in-hand manipulation?

2. *Teachers:* Think about the children in your classrooms who do not have a well-established hand preference. How does this influence their ability to complete refined fine motor, writing, or art projects? What kinds of materials do you offer in the classroom or therapy room to enhance fine motor development and complementary hand use (both hands simultaneously engaged in a task, although each hand plays a different role, such as opening a jar)? How can you arrange the classroom environment to allow for more "floor time" for natural postural adjustment, and more "tummy time" (lying on the floor) for arm/shoulder stability and the differentiation of hand use? Review and add to the list of ways to facilitate hand preference for the "switching" child. How do you adjust task demand for the "switching" child?

3. *Team:* discuss the methods you use to teach pencil grasp in kindergarten, first, second, and third grades. Review the variations of pencil grasp. Review and add to the list of ways to facilitate a more mature pencil grasp. How do you adjust task demand for the child with an immature grasp that creates a barrier to performance?

4. Play some of the haptic exercises described in Chapter 3. How do they enhance learning in math? Literacy? Think of three additional haptic games.

5. Discuss the various ways that drawing is incorporated for learning in your classroom or therapy room. How do you use drawing activities to facilitate children's oral language ability and the conveyance of meaning? Name three ways to scaffold drawing ability.

CHAPTER 4
When Little Hands Write

1. The author has referred to the highly integrated nature of handwriting and to the vital need for collaboration in discovering barriers to the writing process. Why is this understanding essential?

2. *Teachers:* Please answer any questions the team may have regarding the definitions or implications of linguistic processes such as phonological awareness, phonemic awareness, rapid automatic naming (RAN), and orthographic knowledge.

3. How are reading and writing related, and why are they often taught concurrently?

4. Review and discuss the recursive processes of writing. What is transcription, and what are the two component processes of transcription? How do the transcription skills relate to writing fluency and compositional quality?

5. The author has stated that a "red flag" should be raised regarding handwriting when children struggle with these linguistic processes. Why? How does RAN relate to printing automaticity? How does orthographic coding relate to printing speed? How does phonemic awareness relate to printing accuracy? What is the relationship between handwriting and spelling? Review the sequence of steps involved in the spelling-to-handwriting process.

6. What is an *allograph*? A *graphic motor pattern*? What might signal instability in the memory or automaticity of the allograph? What is the importance of establishing automaticity of allograph and graphic motor pattern? What are the implications for handwriting?

7. How do fine motor abilities constrain handwriting in the primary grades? Do pencil grasp and hand preference influence writing legibility, speed, or endurance? Why does the author continue to support explicit instruction for pencil grasp?

8. What are the nine basic forms (beginning with the vertical line) that determine readiness for formal handwriting instruction? When do most children master the ability to copy these forms? When is the ini-

tiation of formal handwriting instruction recommended by the author? How does this recommendation affect your current instructional schedule?

9. How can the kindergarten teacher prepare children for handwriting prior to the inception of formal instruction? How can the reading–writing link of literacy development be addressed prior to the inception of formal handwriting instruction?

10. Review the two lines of research regarding the relationship between writing and drawing. Are these skills distinct in development, or does one gradually emerge from the other? How can drawing support literacy development?

11. Role play the *five-step handwriting process* described by the author. What is the rationale for finger tracing? Random practice?

12. The author describes the need for a *preventive*, rather than solely a *remedial*, approach to handwriting. What is the difference and how is a preventive approach developed by the education team?

CHAPTER 5
Seven Senses in School

1. What are the *far senses*? *Near senses*? How can you balance the benefits of all sensation in the classroom?

2. What is the definition of *adaptive response*? How can a response be purposeful but not adaptive?

3. What is the basis for Dr. A. Jean Ayres's theory of sensory integration? To what does the term *sensory processing* refer?

4. What are the three response patterns of *sensory modulation disorder* (SMD)? What is being *modulated*?

5. What can cause arousal to escalate immediately for the child who is overresponsive? What can cause a gradual escalation of arousal? What are some of the behavioral characteristics of the overresponsive child?

6. What does *hypervigilance* mean, and how is this state different from distractibility?

7. Why is the overresponsive child likely to become aggressive? Why might he or she withdraw? Why might the overresponsive child become rigid and inflexible?

8. How can the classroom or school environments support or create barriers to learning for the overresponsive child?

9. How can you support the academic and social engagement of the overresponsive child?

10. Describe some characteristics of the underresponsive child. Discuss environmental, academic, and social strategies that support adaptive response and occupational performance for this child.

11. Describe some characteristics of the sensory-seeking child. Discuss environmental, academic, and social strategies that support adaptive response and occupational performance for this child.

12. How is a sensory diet similar to a nutritional diet? Why does the author indicate that sensation through *any* sensory channel can be used to appropriately support any child with SMD? How can movement be alerting versus calming? How can touch be alerting versus calming? Sound? Taste?

13. Review the Chapter 5 Appendix (see page 136). Which of these strategies or materials have been recommended for children in your classroom? What is their rationale? What is the expected benefit of each?

14. How can you apply the principles of sensory processing to the development of curricular strategies, methods, and educational environments for all children?

CHAPTER 6
The Knowledge-Sharing Team in Action

1. Role play some of the "writing without writing" activities. How do they contribute to the automaticity of handwriting in the writing process, even though the activities are "pencil-less"?

2. Arrange an in-service or seminar on dynamic assessment. How can your education team move toward this model?

3. How does collaborative knowledge sharing by the education team lead to a balance of assumptions regarding the potential contributors of at-risk affect, behavior, or occupational performance in students?

4. How has an understanding of the interplay among student factors, environmental components, and task demand contributed to your ability to design and evaluate effective curricular activities? How has it broadened your capacity to evaluate student performance and performance barriers?

5. How has the information in this book influenced your perspective on the need to engage in knowledge sharing among education team members?

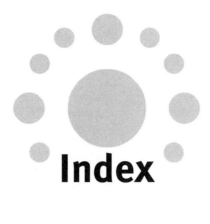

Index

Page references followed by *f*, *t*, or *n* indicate figures, tables, or footnotes, respectively.

Early arrival or dismissal, 141
Earphones, noise-reduction, 123
Education, 7–8
  brain-based, 26–30
  cognition and, 25
  sensory diet, 130–131
Education for All Handicapped Children
    Act of 1975 (PL 94-142), 10
Education teams
  collaboration of, 146–150
  questions to ask, 146–147
  study guide for, 171–176
Educational environment(s), 4–7
Educational performance
  components of, 1, 2f
  factors that affect movement automaticity
    and, 32–33
Educational relevance, 11
Educational theory, 7
Educationalizing, 15
Effectiveness, 92–94
Efficiency, 92–94
Empathy disorders, 44
Engagement, social and academic
  and overresponsive children, 120–122
  and sensory-seeking behavior, 127–128
  and underresponsive children, 125
English language, 77
English language arts (ELA), 18
Environment(s), 4–7
  assessment and, 155
  classroom modifications, 38–42, 137–138
  components of, 5–6
  and movement–learning link, 150
  and overresponsive children, 118–120
  questions to ask about, 148–149
  and sensory-seeking children, 126–127
  and underresponsive children, 124–125
Epistemology, 7
Essential Academic Learning Requirements
    (EALRs), 18–19
Exercise(s), 101
Explicit instruction, 95
Eye, language by, 76

Fans, 141
Far senses, 47, 110–111
Fearfulness, 118
Finger pushups, 101

Finger tracing, 94
Fitness, 30
Five-step handwriting process, 93, 94
Frames of reference, 11–12
Functional ability, 31
Furniture, 38–42, 136–137, 138

Games
  Clap the Space, 153
  Concentration, 151, 154
  Follow the Arrows, 152
  haptic recognition games, 65–66
  Head or Belt, 152
  idea generation, 154
  Letter, Sound, Stroke, 152
  line orientation, 153
  Musical Chairs, 151
  Out to Dry, 153
  Phoneme to Grapheme, 153
  punctuation, 154
  Red Light, Green Light, 150
  Show Me the Way, 152
  Silly Sounds, 152
  spelling, 153
  for stabilizing allographs, 150–151
  for stabilizing graphic motor patterns,
    151–153
  Tall, Small or Diver? 151
  Teacher's Mistake, 153
  What Am I? 151
  Where's the Arrow? 152
  Which Direction?, 151
  Who's Getting Tired? 153
  word spacing, 153
  word usage, 154
  The Writing Train, 152
Gardner, Howard, 25
Gesture, 28–29
Girls, 37
Global human figures, 71–72
Grade Level Expectations (GLEs), 18–19
Graffiti centers, 39
Graphemes, 76
Graphemic buffers, 83, 84f
Graphic motor patterns, 83, 84f, 151–153
Graphic production, 71–72
Grasp
  strategies to help children grasp scissors,
    63–64, 64f